SCARRED

# Scarred

*A Feminist Journey Through Pain*

L. Ayu Saraswati

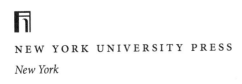

NEW YORK UNIVERSITY PRESS

*New York*

NEW YORK UNIVERSITY PRESS
New York
www.nyupress.org

Library of Congress Cataloging-in-Publication Data
Names: Saraswati, L. Ayu, author.
Title: Scarred : a feminist journey through pain / L. Ayu Saraswati.
Description: New York : New York University Press, [2023] |
Includes bibliographical references and index.
Identifiers: LCCN 2022036289 | ISBN 9781479817078 (hardback) |
ISBN 9781479817092 (paperback) | ISBN 9781479817108 (ebook) |
ISBN 9781479817115 (ebook other)
Subjects: LCSH: Women—Psychology. | Women—Travel. | Pain—Psychological aspects.
Classification: LCC HQ1206 .S26 2023 | DDC 155.3/33—dc23/eng/20220809
LC record available at https://lccn.loc.gov/2022036289

New York University Press books are printed on acid-free paper, and their binding materials
are chosen for strength and durability. We strive to use environmentally responsible suppliers
and materials to the greatest extent possible in publishing our books.

Manufactured in the United States of America

10 9 8 7 6 5 4 3 2 1

Also available as an ebook

# CONTENTS

# AUTHOR'S NOTE

During the pandemic, every time I saw someone in the media mingling freely with others without a mask, I would cringe. I projected my own fear onto them. I was worried for their health. I do not want the readers of this book to have a similar reaction. Hence, this note. The travels in this book took place between May 2017 and August 2018, more than a year before the pandemic hit. Hopefully, by the time this book is published, we will be living in a world where wild travels and nonawkward hugs are possible. This note is meant to create a pause, a gentle transitional space for the readers to mentally return to that prepandemic world. I hope cringing is unnecessary, except in those moments when I share too much information.

I have created pseudonyms for people mentioned in this book. Certain omissions in regard to people, places, and events have been made without altering the integrity of the story. Data and links presented in this book are accurate as of the time I write this book in 2020. For readers who would like to see some pictures from my travels, they are accessible on my website, drsaraswati.com.

On my writing style: I deliberately choose a style that crosses multiple genres and hopefully reaches not only academic but also general audiences. For readers who may find the theoretical part of this book tedious, I invite them to dip in and out of the text as they wish and "choose their own adventure," so to speak. For readers in academia, I invite them to read the end notes—the space where I let my nerdy self shine. I live simultaneously in academic and nonacademic spaces, the worlds of theories and of stories. Sometimes theory is part of the story; sometimes it wants to show up as distinct from the story. I let it be.

My only hope is that I have written the practical and theoretical parts of the book clearly enough for *all* readers to grasp the essence of this book. It aims to shed light on important questions in our lives that we need to think more carefully about, so we can live with pain differently, in a way that is more life sustaining, humane, and feminist (social justice oriented). I wish the readers a plentiful and delightful journey, with this book, and in life. Always.

1

# All about Pain

Perhaps Billy Joel was right: Vienna waits for me. Sitting in the corner of Café Central in Vienna, Austria, my lips full of a smile and whipped cream from the Viennese-style iced coffee, I delighted in the ordinary wonder of being alive. The place itself was hectic, with tourists and locals alike waiting in a long line before finally scoring a spot. Yet, the smells of strong espresso and sweet cakes, from glossy apricot dome to raspberry harmony, neatly lined up behind glass, creating a spectacle of delectable color, gently halted the movement of time. In that moment of satiating quietude, my heart became still. After days and nights of being buoyed by Vienna's gorgeous gardens and stimulating scenes, from art to Mozart, I felt that somehow my pain had slowly waned. I wondered, *Could travel really heal?*

After traveling to twenty countries (Indonesia, France, Czech Republic, Portugal, Germany, England, Montenegro, Nepal, Spain, Iceland, Australia, New Zealand, Costa Rica, Canada, Hungary, Austria, Japan, Peru, Ecuador, and Singapore) in one year—or, one year and two and a half months to be exact—I still cannot answer with utmost certainty whether travel can really heal. To pretend to know the answer is to betray the very core of what it means to be human: that we are all different. Our bodies are different. Our responses to pain are different. Our traveling styles are also different. Any attempt to come up with a formulaic answer that prescribes a way of traveling that can heal us all will inevitably dismiss the varieties of our genetic and psychic makeup.

What I *can* say, and what I will share in this book, is that there are four things that traveling to all of these places in one year has made me think about. Reflecting on them deeply has helped me shift my relationship with pain. It is my hope that the readers of this book can use these main questions as a launchpad from which to begin to meditate on these four issues, so they, too, can take their own journey to explore what a nourishing relationship with pain would look like for them.[1]

In a nutshell, *Scarred: A Feminist Journey Through Pain* tells a story of how we can carry pain in a way that is more humane, life sustaining, enchanting, and feminist (social justice oriented). It begins with a simple premise: we all carry pain in our lives. We just carry it in different ways. Because our quality of life depends on how we carry pain, we therefore need to explore other and better ways of carrying it. This book thus points to the key questions that can help us shift our relationship with pain.

The first question, "How can I perceive differently?" (chapter 3), invites us to look closely at a very intimate part of ourselves: our minds—the thoughts and perceptions that are going on in our heads as we experience an event. But here, I am not interested in the neoliberal idea that tells us that to be pain free, we need to change our attitude, or worse, to "just think positive" and dismiss our real-life issues.[2] Instead, I am more intrigued by how the personal collides and colludes with the structural, an intersection I approach by meditating on these questions: What does our society teach us about how to perceive? Is our perception "docile"? Does it further create pain in our lives? How can we perceive in ways that do not provoke even more pain and that liberate us from the shackles of societal gendered norms? Put simply, How can we perceive differently?

Second, following an investigation of the mind, I shift our attention to the body (chapter 4). Changing our mind/perception, no matter how radical it may be, will not be enough. This chapter thus provides us with one example of how we can process pain by working *with* our body and *without* the story (thereby bypassing the limitations of the mind) so we can engage with and transcend pain at a deeper level. The second important question this book asks is thus, How can I work with my body to process pain?

Next, I invite the readers to explore embodied practices that they can do every day to carry pain differently (chapter 5). Shifting the mind and working with the body are indeed necessary, yet, we need to do something every day to shift our relationship with pain. I thus propose a daily embodied practice that I call "feminist enchantment." This practice connects the mind and the body with their cultural and material milieus (the physical spaces within which the body moves), and aims to cultivate habits that can take us to moments of enchantment. Another central question raised in this book is therefore, How can I practice feminist enchantment in my everyday life?

Lastly, for the fourth area of reflection, I expand the conversation about the milieu to include the nation-state (chapter 6). After turning the gaze inward toward ourselves (our mind, body, and embodied daily practice), we need to turn the gaze outward and contemplate how where we live contributes to how we experience, express, and address the pain in our lives. Remember, *pain is never only personal.* It is also social, structural, and political. We therefore need to ask, What programs and policies does our government have that can help us carry pain in a more life-sustaining way? It is thus inevitable and necessary that we ask, How does where I live matter to my pain?

These pain-shifting questions aim to nudge the readers to go toward certain directions of inquiry, so they, too, can find the answers *for themselves.* This book does not tell the readers that this is the way to heal. In fact, if by the end of the book the readers ask themselves, "How can *I* live with pain differently?" then this book has succeeded in accomplishing its modest goal.

The book's main goal is to invite readers to ponder these questions, which would propel them to shift their relationship with pain, without necessarily having to travel the world.[3] I recognize that traveling the world is a privilege (I discuss this in chapter 2), and if what I propose is that healing is predicated upon one's ability to travel the world, then, this book already fails before it even begins. The traveling matters in *theorizing*, but is not necessary in *healing*. In other words, I consider traveling as important in thinking about the theories and the questions raised in this book (i.e., traveling as a method—hence, the "transnational feminist autoethnography" method I discuss in chapter 2), but not necessarily in the process of healing itself.

It follows, then, that this book does more than just propose the important questions that can help us shift our relationship with pain. This book also makes (1) a methodological contribution, by offering a method that I call "transnational feminist autoethnography"; and (2) a theoretical contribution, by providing a new meaning of pain as a transnational feminist object—I will explain this in the next section.

## Reframing Our Relationship with Pain: Pain as a Transnational Feminist Object

Let us begin with an obvious and necessary question: What is pain? The International Association for the Study of Pain (IASP) defines pain as "an unpleasant sensory and emotional experience associated with actual or potential tissue damage, or described in terms of such damage."[4] Pain can also be seen as a perception (relying on the mind and emotion), and not a sensation (relying more on the nervous system).[5] In the medical world, injury to the body does not always cause pain, and the intensity of pain is not always in a direct relationship to the level of damage in the body.[6] Pain is thus not a self-explanatory feeling, and why it manifests cannot always be explained.[7]

In this book, however, I have no interest in reducing pain to a physical and/or affective manifestation alone, as doing so would disregard power, various social constructions of difference (race, gender, and so forth), and sites where pain is valued (such as in narratives of martyrs).[8] Instead, I want to rely on and work with feminist theorist Gloria Anzaldúa's understanding of pain.

With fervor, Anzaldúa wrote that "pain is the way of life."[9] As unforgiving as this conviction may sound, there is something soothing about this way of framing our relationship with pain. Pain is neither good nor bad, neither "celebrated [n]or rejected," but rather, is "expansive, leading to the creation of new forms of being."[10] Pain is not something that we should deny but rather something to return to faithfully.[11] In this spirit of not denying pain, Anzaldúa even argues that our ultimate goal should not simply be healing but instead "making meaning of pain."[12]

I take Anzaldúa's invitation a step further by not only making new meanings of pain but also offering new ways of relating to pain and theorizing *with* (rather than just *about*) pain. I use "pain" as a *theoretical hook* on which all forms of trauma, suffering, not feeling/being well, being hurt, and being wounded (all of which may originate in the physical or psychological—not mutually exclusive) are all cautiously hung.

I want to tinker here with the idea that pain can be a way of a *feminist* life. Feminism often relies on the "exhibition of pain" to provide proof that harm has been done to women and to demand change.[13] Theorist bell hooks highlights the importance of pain by framing it as something that we need to "remember . . . because . . . true resistance begins with people confronting pain, whether it's theirs or somebody else's, and wanting to do something to change it. . . . That is what connects us—our awareness that we know [pain], have known it, or will know it again."[14] Pain is central in feminist narrative and has served as a platform for its activism, as a site at which to connect and resist.[15]

I build on this relationship between pain and feminism further by offering a new model of relating to pain as a transnational feminist object—as something that we *carry* with us to help us understand something (the "X") differently.[16] As a transnational feminist object that I carry during my transnational travels, I frame pain more specifically as *an orienting tool* that triggers us to move away (in this context, transnationally) from something that is wounding us, and as *an anamorphic apparatus* that makes visible matters (e.g., how power and gender ideology work) that were previously hidden. Let us unpack all of these important concepts below.

*Pain as Something That We Carry*

We do not experience pain as itself. We experience pain as *how we carry it*. We thus need to carry pain in a way that holds the integrity of the pain as well as the integrity of our own body. To honor the integrity of the pain, we must first consider pain as an integral part of bodily construction, but not part of the body itself. I want to draw here from women's studies scholar Leigh Gilmore, who frames pain as an actant (an actor that can "modify" other actors) that shares a (or "our") body to propose a new metaphor for pain.[17]

I argue that pain is to the body what its shell is to a hermit crab.[18] For a hermit crab, its shell is an integral part of its everyday living system; however, it cannot grow its own shell. When it outgrows its shell, it has to find an abandoned shell from another creature. Similarly, pain (not the actual tumor or wound itself) is an integral part of the living system of that body/organism, but it remains "exterior" or external to the body.

This ambiguous and ambivalent site of pain and its relationship to one's body has been articulated by different scholars. Feminist theorist Sara Ahmed gets at this sentiment by pointing out how pain "is not a part of me, even though it is in my body that I feel it."[19] For philosophy of medicine professor Richard Zaner, pain is an "alien presence" in one's body.[20] For feminist philosopher Elaine Scarry, "Even though [pain] occurs within oneself, it is at once identified as 'not oneself,' 'not me,' as something so alien that it must right now be gotten rid of."[21] All of these articulations (including mine) thus hint at pain's ambiguous relationship to the body: *as an integral part of the living body, but not internal to it.*

I also find the hermit crab shell to be an apt metaphor for pain's protective functions. Pain, too, works to protect the human body and is necessary for our survival.[22] As philosopher Fredrik Svenaeus points out, "Pain appears to be a kind of signal of distress: It hurts, do something about it, stop moving, go to the doctor, etc."[23] For writer and artist Thyrza Goodeve, "Pain, whether one describes it as a sensation, an emotion, or merely a warning system, is a response to damage. . . . Although terrible in feeling, pain is a good thing. It lets us know there is something that can—and should be—fixed."[24] Drawing from these arguments, I, too, consider pain as protective and productive, as it warns us of the perceived dangers that threaten the equilibrium of our well-being,[25] and allows us to generate new knowledge based on our pain inquiry. Thus, although I consider pain as a transnational feminist *object*, I write into pain a sense of subjectivity/agency nonetheless. I cast pain as a protagonist, playing a leading role, whose voice and virtue can orient us into more subversive ways of thinking, theorizing, and living.

The shell metaphor is also useful in illustrating how one "carries" pain (the shell) with one's body. As something that is exterior to the body, pain is carried with our body. If pain is something that we carry, then, we can figure out a better way to carry it, or find a new shell when the old one no longer fits. Here is what I propose: because how we carry pain is socially constructed—every family, culture, and nation may teach us to carry pain differently—we need to understand how the body is taught to carry pain in gendered (as an intersectional construction) ways, and how the operationalization of gender ideologies produces pain in the first place. This is an important endeavor, considering how the body in some foundational texts about pain, including Scarry's work, for instance, is not necessarily marked as gendered. With this book, I want to offer several ways to unlearn old ways of carrying pain and cultivate new ways (cognitively, affectively, physiologically, phenomenologically, etc.) that are more life sustaining to us. To return to the hermit crab shell metaphor one more time, we thus need to find a new shell that may "fit" and serve us better as we carry pain in our lives.

### Pain as a Transnational Feminist Object I: As an Orienting Tool

Pain orients us. Pain can function as a map we use to achieve a good life, by doing what we can do to avoid and eliminate pain in our lives.[26] In this sense, pain can be considered as an orienting tool. As a system of orientation, pain is an *unreliable* orienting tool. It tells us to move away from something, yet it does not tell us where to move to/toward.

For instance, Nancy Gardner Prince, an early-nineteenth-century Black American traveler, noted that she left the United States because it was making her anxious and worn out due to racial discrimination and having to provide for her family/siblings: "After seven years of anxiety and toil, I made up my mind to leave my country."[27] The women of Girlfriend Tours International (GFT) (mostly African American women) also had to "momentarily leave the spaces that many argue should make them happy—their families, their homes in their native country, and their jobs" and travel abroad in their pursuit of happiness.[28] That these women of color find transnational travel or relocation as their saving grace signals how race and gender intersect in structuring transnational movements of bodies. In a similar vein, I, too, a woman of color, wanted that experience. I wanted to find other spaces where my pain could feel distant, stranger, and foreign to me. I wanted to turn pain into a foreign object and experience its foreignness. Perhaps, then, I could carry and relate to pain differently.

I knew that I wanted to leave Hawai'i, my perceived site of wounding, but I did not know where exactly to go. When I set out to travel for one entire year, I did not plan to visit twenty countries. I was open to whatever countries I would end up visiting as a way of being curious about the unknown. Except for the specific countries I had to go to because I had workshops there (Indonesia, Peru, Japan, Spain), because I wanted to visit friends and family (Indonesia, Canada, Australia, Germany), or because I had it on my bucket list (Iceland), I did not know what other countries I would visit. I used the app Skyscanner to choose my next destination. This app allowed me to type in "everywhere" instead of a specific city of arrival. The app then provided me with a list of possible places to visit, from the cheapest to the most expensive. For instance, when I was staying at my brother's place in Fürth/Nuremberg, the city of Kotor, Montenegro, appeared as one of the cheapest places to fly to. Since Montenegro had been on my list of places to go, it was an easy decision for me to make my dream come true. At other times, I would find cheap places to fly to, but not stay at. Dublin, Ireland, for instance, was a city I would like to visit, but since I could not find an affordable accommodation there, I eventually skipped it. It was budgetary limitations that shaped the decision for my destinations, rather than the pain itself.

As an unreliable orienting tool, pain can be *disorienting*. It creates a necessary pause (to reorient) and a recognition of the direction we assumed to be correct, and this is what makes us question all the ways we orient ourselves (questioning who we are: our essence, our sense of the world, and our life purpose). In this sense, pain as a(n) (dis)orienting tool can be chaotic and create chaos. Carrying pain as an orienting tool also means that we are aware of where and how pain moves across nations, what pain moves, and what moves pain. As I will detail throughout the chapters of this book, pain has the capacity to push us toward nonlinear journeys of unbecoming, unlearning, and undoing. I am intrigued, therefore, to explore what this (dis)orienting capacity of pain can do to our relationship with and experience of carrying pain in our lives, and, of course, to our feminist theorizing about pain in general.

### Pain as a Transnational Feminist Object II: As an Anamorphic Apparatus

In travel writing,[29] it is not a coincidence—indeed, it is a common trope—that writers use books to reflect on their lives (as "mirror events").[30] Here, books function as "reflexive and anamorphic eyes," providing the writers with "a structure within which one can think more critically and objectively about one's role as a traveler."[31] If in travel writing, books function as a structure within which to reflect and think, in this book, I use pain as a transnational feminist object that I carry and travel with, to reflect, think, and theorize: pain is my anamorphic apparatus. Wherever I go I bring my pain with me.

"Anamorphosis" is a term often found in art and refers to "a perspective that is present but cannot be perceived unless the viewer knows how to look."[32] Worded differently, "An anamorphic image is one that can only be interpreted when viewed from a particular angle or through a transforming optical device like a mirror."[33] A famous painting by Hans Holbein the Younger, *The Ambassadors*, for instance, has an image of a skull in it. The skull, however, can only be seen when the viewer is looking at the painting from the right angle. Otherwise, the skull would appear as "splodge."[34] Another example is letters painted in an artwork in reverse, so that we need a mirror to read what the letters spell.

Thus, pain as an anamorphic lens means that pain functions as a transforming optical device that makes visible things previously unseen or registered as sublime. It then allows us to understand things differently and theorize about different things. For instance, in this book, without pain as an anamorphic apparatus that I carry during my travels, I would not have been able to theorize and propose the concept of emotional contract to chart the different relationships each nation-state has with its citizens and their pain (see chapter 6). Nor would I have been able to understand and challenge the docile ways in which we perceive that may cause us pain (chapter 3), find ways to bypass language in processing pain (chapter 4), or evoke enchantment as an antidote to pain (chapter 5).[35]

Pain as an anamorphic apparatus thus reconfigures our ways of seeing and knowing the world—it is an episteme.[36] In this book, I frame pain as a means of knowing and telling different, more subversive, and feminist theories/stories. Employing pain as an anamorphic apparatus, I seek to decode the stories that pain tells us of how to live our lives, what kind of life we desire and deem worthy of living, what life choices we make when we have a different relationship with pain, what it allows us to know, what it connects us with, and what it makes possible.

My conceptualization of pain as a transnational feminist object that we carry during our travels challenges previous articulations of pain as negative and nonreferential (as "something contained within itself . . . [and] . . . within the boundaries of an individual's body . . . because pain does not reference anything but itself").[37] As a transnational feminist object that we carry, I argue, pain is both productive and referential. Here, I do not mean pain as "productive" in the neoliberal sense of the word: that the person in pain needs to be productive by finding ways to heal themselves, to think positively in the midst of pain, or to turn pain into something "good." Rather, by considering pain as productive, I want to highlight the usefulness of pain (i.e., as an anamorphic apparatus) in producing knowledge. Pain produces knowledge.

I consider pain as referential in the sense that pain refers to the ecology (which includes human and nonhuman, and material and nonmaterial) that causes that very pain to begin with. That is, the pain we carry with our bodies is not contained within itself, but rather, it points us to the sick ecology that needs transforming. Bodies may "carry within them the symptoms of a sick world."[38] This is why traveling, the shifting of ecologies, may help us contextualize and conceptualize pain differently. Thus, although the questions I pose may seem to be registered at the individual level (e.g., as "my" perception, "my" body, etc.), they are not solely about the self. Rather, these questions simultaneously point to the structure and the ecology that create pain and that need to be changed and challenged. In this way, to process pain is to also work toward social change.

One final and critical note of clarification for this section: I am often asked whether the pain I am analyzing is psychological *or* physiological. For the purpose of this book, I refuse to subscribe to this duality of pain.[39] I recognize that this very question is rooted in the limited Western understanding of pain that separates the mind from the body, emotional from physical pain, and that fails to see the intricate flow and interconnection between emotional and physical pain, or how one is expressed through the other.[40] I thus treat pain in this book as a site at which to pause and ponder, rather than put an order or a border around pain.

## An Overview of the Book

Suzanne Bost ends her article "Gloria Anzaldúa's Mestiza Pain: Mexican Sacrifice, Chicana Embodiment, and Feminist Politics" with these powerful words: "Complacency feeds status quo; pain makes trouble."[41] Her insight inspires and illuminates how I approach pain in this book: as a transnational feminist object (an orienting tool and anamorphic apparatus) to make trouble and theorize with, and as a lens to see what (feminist) trouble pain could create.

At its theoretical core, this book asks, If feminist theories aim to improve women's (and people's) lives, then how can they be useful in answering one of life's most troubling questions of what to do with pain? How do feminist theories help us shift our relationship with pain—to our experiencing, expressing, and engaging with pain? What does feminist theory do *to* and *with* pain? How does pain function as a site of theorizing feminisms? And how does examining pain help us further feminist theories?

In answering these complex questions, and deeply and critically interrogating the relationship between pain and feminism, and its implications for feminist theorizing and feminist living, this book offers a new approach by making a transnational feminist autoethnographic intervention (based on my traveling to twenty countries) into the ways in which we theorize pain. This book also proposes a fresh perspective on pain by framing it as a transnational feminist object that we *carry* rather than embody (i.e., we feel, we have) or identify with (i.e., we are) during our movement across national borders, which, in turn, can help us understand something, the "X" that we are analyzing, differently.

In chapter 2, "On the Method of Transnational Feminist Autoethnography," I delight in detailing the method that I developed and employed for this book, "transnational feminist autoethnography." I make explicit its genealogies—a merging of autoethnography and transnational feminism—and how travel or movement across national borders is at the methodological center of its theory and knowledge production.

In chapters 3–6, as mentioned in the beginning of this chapter, I move through each of the key questions posed in the book. I interrogate the mind/perception (chapter 3); the body (chapter 4); the embodied daily practice—contextualized within its milieus (chapter 5); and finally (by way of expanding that milieu to include) the nation-state (chapter 6). In this way, each chapter is built on and meant to push further the points articulated in the previous one. When read linearly, these chapters are meant to take the readers deeper and deeper into the process of understanding and transcending pain that they (or other people) have carried throughout their lives. These chapters are also intended to provide examples of how *I* address these questions in my life. Hopefully, by reading my stories, the readers will then be able to better explore these questions, and find the answers and practices that work *for them*.

In chapter 3, "How Can I Perceive Differently?," I use my experiences of attending a women-only retreat in Costa Rica to show the processes of how we are trained to perceive in ways that support the dominant power and that may hurt us—I call this "docile perception." Here, I follow the logic that if perception shapes the experience of pain, then that experience will inevitably change when we shift our perception and understanding of perception. I thus propose that we cultivate a different, more defiant mode of perceiving—one that rejects, resists, and rebels against the dominant ideology, and one that does not keep us in the cycle of being in pain.

In chapter 4, "How Can I Work with My Body to Process Pain?," I shift my attention from the mind to the body. I share my experiences at a meditation ashram in Nepal to illustrate how the existing mode of processing pain—by expressing it (in writing, speech, etc.) in ways that others or the self can understand (that is, via discourses, including feminist discourses)—has limited us in going deeper into our pain, in resurfacing our emotions, especially those emotions that are registered precognitively, and in transforming them. I thus suggest that we work with/as the body and without the story to process our pain.

In chapter 5, "How Can I Practice Feminist Enchantment in My Everyday Life?," I reflect on my travels to Ecuador, Spain, Iceland, and Montenegro to introduce an embodied daily practice that I call "feminist enchantment," and explain its three core practices (i.e., forgetting, embodying the erotic, and being playful). As a concept and a practice, feminist enchantment connects the mind, the body, and the materiality of one's physical and cultural milieus,[42] to push us toward a way of carrying pain that is more humane, enchanting, life sustaining, and feminist.

Chapter 6, "How Does Where I Live Matter to My Pain?," is inspired by my travels to New Zealand, Iceland, and Indonesia. Comparing these countries to the United States, I offer an alternative perspective in examining pain: one that recasts the nation-state as playing an important role in shaping its citizens' experiences of their pain and well-being. Individuals can only do so much to address the pain in their lives (i.e., working with the mind/body/surrounding); they also need structural support from the government. When countries consider the well-being of their citizens as a priority and as a form of recognition that the root cause of pain is oftentimes structural and political, they will have what I call an "emotional contract" as part of their social contract with their citizens.[43]

In the final chapter, chapter 7, "Home(ostasis) Is Where the Heart Is . . . Healed," I end with a meditation on home to offer a sense of *completion*, rather than a conclusion. All travels must come to an end, and so must this book. The final chapter, written in the form of vignettes, proposes that it is homeostasis, rather than home per se, that is a site of healing.

As an academic book, *Scarred* indulges in a conversation that traverses diverse theoretical terrain and intersects various inter/disciplinary locations, from transnational feminist theory to travel studies to pain studies to philosophy to sociology and to anthropology, among other fields. It mixes and merges different genres and forms of writing, from memoir to academic text.[44] It explores the personal, epistemological, ideological, theoretical, transnational, emotional/affective, and material dimensions of pain experience.

This book thus aims to intervene in the fields of (1) autoethnography (by proposing the method that I call "transnational feminist autoethnography"); (2) phenomenology and embodiment (by focusing on how bodies-in-pain travel); (3) travel studies and transnational feminist studies (by examining and using the lens of pain while traveling); and (4) pain studies (by reframing pain as an object that moves and is carried across nations and does particular ideological-emotional work; by theorizing pain from a transnational feminist perspective and as a transnational feminist object that can help us better understand a wide range of subjects from perception to enchantment, etc.; and by exploring different forms of pain embodiment, expression, and experience). In these ways, this book renders pain as both a powerful trope and a materiality of power that allows us to chart how power produces and operates through pain (chapters 3 and 6) and how pain is embodied and embedded in power relations (chapters 4 and 5).

At a more practical level, this book invites readers to think these larger questions: What different choices in life would they dare to make, had they not been taught that pain is something to avoid and be gotten rid of? And if pain is a way of life and here to stay, how can they carry and relate to it differently? (The book's four areas of reflection indeed aim to invite readers to explore and specifically answer the latter question.) I hope this book can help us find new ways of thinking, experiencing, and carrying pain in our lives: ones that support and sustain us from the very nourishing core of our being.

2

# On the Method of Transnational Feminist Autoethnography

My personal experiences shaped how I came to know what I know, my episteme.

I was born and raised in Jakarta, Indonesia. I then moved to the United States in 1999 to pursue graduate education in Chicago, Illinois, and then College Park, Maryland. In the United States, I began to learn and have the experiences of what it meant to live as a woman of color in a white-male-dominated society. Moving to the United States shook and shocked (as it should) my twenty-two-year-old naïve self, a Javanese ciswoman who was accustomed to living in a society where Javanese ethnicity was privileged. Not knowing how to reorient and position myself in the new country, I internalized racism to the point of avoiding going to certain public white spaces/restaurants, where I was often treated differently. I eventually became depressed and sought professional help, including from psychologists and psychiatrists.

My transnational move afforded me the experiences and, through university classes, the critical lens for my research. I was then able to see racism/colorism/sexism in Indonesia from different perspectives. It is not a surprise that my dissertation, first book, and early articles examined precisely these issues: racism/colorism/sexism in transnational Indonesia.

Because transnationalism has become a key framework in my analyses, I wanted to make the connection among the personal, the epistemological, and the transnational stronger and clearer in this book. I wanted to turn the gaze inward toward how *I*, an Indonesian/Asian woman academic currently living in the United States, grappled, struggled, and worked with pain—pain that stemmed from patriarchy—in my own life.

This book has two main methodological goals. First, I want to illustrate how the personal can be epistemological: a way to systematically know, theorize, and, eventually, transcend our ways of knowing and living in this world. It is a feminist move to value women's personal narratives and emotions as legitimate areas of study in academia.[1] In this way, the work of autoethnographer Carolyn Ellis is significant in that it considers both autobiography and emotions important in a culture that since the nineteenth century has marked them as feminine and therefore not valuable.[2] By using autoethnography, I attempt to revalue both women's writings about the self and emotions, particularly of pain, and women's personal narratives as crucial for knowledge production, including in academia.

Second, I aim to contribute to the specific methodological field of autoethnography, by merging it with transnational feminism—a method that I call "transnational feminist autoethnography."[3] In the act of naming this method, I ascend to the tasks of "liberating" and "naming and claiming" a theoretical approach, which author, activist, and professor Nadine Naber asserts that we as women of color need to do.[4] Rather than trying to force ourselves to fit into an existing theoretical framework that was not written for or by us (let alone talk about our experiences), I want to chart a methodological space where our experiences, our writings, and our ways of thinking/knowing/living matter and are valued.

By proposing a transnational feminist autoethnography method, I also hope to enrich the what and how of the research process, as it uses personal experiences, travels, nodes, crossroads, and sites-in-between as methods and spaces to produce theories about the self and power relationships in a transnational context. A discussion on traveling as research, and then on transnational feminism, may therefore be helpful, before I immerse the readers into the essentials of all that transnational feminist autoethnographic research and writing may entail.

## Traveling as Research

In her book *My Travels around the World* Egyptian physician, author, and feminist activist Nawal El Saadawi wrote, "My face always looks more beautiful in aeroplane mirrors than it does in the mirror at home or in any other mirror in the country. I don't know: do my features change simply by crossing borders, or are aeroplane mirrors of better quality?"[5] Her quirky and witty question captures the pertinent research questions raised in this book: What does the body actually do when it crosses national borders? Does the materiality of the body shift when it travels and inhabits new spaces, thereby causing the body to carry pain in a different way—if so, how and why? Or, is it one's *perception* of one's body that changes when it moves across borders? What is it about traveling that allows the body or one's perception of the body (or of one's self) to shift? Specifically, and most importantly for this book, how and why do the ways in which one relates to or carries pain change when one travels across the world?

In this book, I use travel purposely to engage with the question of *how to do things with pain* and provide us with different modes of relating to pain. I build on works that see travel and holidays as "healing,"[6] and consider traveling as a site where we can navigate and renegotiate our relationship with pain. To return to the hermit crab metaphor of the previous chapter, travel may help us acquire a new shell, so we can carry pain in a more comfortable and life-sustaining way.

I approach travel as an embodied act, and incorporate "embodiment and affect" in my analysis.[7] This means that I pay attention to the materiality (the flesh, the physical, the tangible) and emotionality of the body and its changing environments during travels. I also interrogate how travel itself can open up spaces of pain: spaces that pain creates, yields, and takes up. I thus follow in the footsteps of scholars of color who ground their analysis in "theory in the flesh"—which emphasizes how the (movement of) body matters in fleshing out experience, and eventually, in theorizing.[8]

Although travel can be used as a tool to distract us from pain,[9] I employ it here as an instrument with which to theorize, translate, and make visible how I might have misunderstood, misplaced, and displaced pain.[10] Traveling allows me to do the work of tracing and putting pain in its place, where it belongs—its "home." I contend that *to heal is to have found a home for the wound*.

Traveling provides us with a different ecology (physical, nonphysical, and beyond) that provokes our body to shift, which in turn may then allow us to process, live with, and carry pain differently. As cancer physician and researcher Siddhartha Mukherjee points out, if we change the body's environment, cancer cells can behave significantly differently.[11] In the field of neurology, scientists have shown that traveling abroad outside one's comfort zone to experience new things, learn a new language, or try new food affects neurons firing and influences "brain plasticity."[12] During travels, the brain's neural pathways that are stimulated by new sounds and smells will then be rewired. Studies show that people who have traveled to more countries tend to be more creative than those who have not; the key here is that the travel needs to be long term—at least four to eight months.[13] This would allow travelers to engage with and be immersed in the local culture.[14] Similarly, as my book points out, traveling transports the body into a new environment, which may trigger the body to behave differently. Traveling can thus function as a "cultural laboratory,"[15] a playground for trying out new identities and ways of relating to others, nature, and even pain.

Two points I want to clarify here. First, there are so many benefits of traveling, as mentioned above, and I would encourage anyone to travel when they can. I remain convinced, however, that traveling abroad is *not* a *necessary* condition for healing. I highlight the importance of traveling to emphasize that traveling/crossing borders matters in this book insofar as it works as a different *method* in producing knowledge about pain (or whatever research question one hopes to answer) but not necessarily in addressing the pain itself. As can be seen from the key questions raised in this book, they do not require the readers to travel the world to answer them.

Second, this book is not a travel guidebook that details each and every country I visited. In fact, there are more countries that did not make it into the pages of this book than those that did. My interest for this book is not in summarizing and scrutinizing how people in/and other countries are different from me/us. Oftentimes, the production of difference in travel writing is problematic, if not downright imperialistic, because it portrays the self as the more evolved and superior hero in the story. Instead, I am more invested in producing new knowledges about pain. When I write stories and theories of travel as they relate to particular countries, they are meant to serve as a *thinking from*, a launchpad to theorize about X. In chapter 6, for example, I am not writing about Iceland or New Zealand per se. My visits to these countries push me to theoretically ponder the different affective modes of governance and what it means for a country to have an emotional contract with its citizens, rather than to describe what the people or the places are like.

## Women and Travel

I sneak in this brief history of women and travel here for my fellow women travelers.[16] Although these days, I often encounter other women who travel solo—they are usually the people I make friends with during my travels—women have not always been able to travel or write about it. Women were excluded from scientific and discovery journeys of the sixteenth and seventeenth centuries, except for in conditions of bondage.[17] They were assigned to the domestic domain.[18] A small number of women did, however, travel and wrote their accounts although those that circulated in public often embody the stereotypical "indomitable eccentric spinsters" narrative figure.[19]

In the second half of the eighteenth century, and throughout the Victorian era, there was an increase in women's travel, which reflected the shifting social meanings of travel as a leisure activity and the phenomenon of "scenic tourism" in Europe.[20] In addition to traveling for pleasure, women at the time also traveled to do missionary work or to join their husbands in the colonies.[21] It is not a surprise, then, that the women's writings that came out of this period often took the form of diaries or letters, such as letters written by Lady Mary Montagu, based on her travels to Constantinople from 1716 to 1718.[22]

During the mid- to late nineteenth century, women (mostly white and privileged) had more opportunities to travel due to modernity.[23] Colonialism provided women from the colonizing countries with access to travel and the ability to become travel writers.[24] Women's travel writing during the colonial period is nonetheless read and produced differently from men's because adventure stories were considered "unfeminine"; women were seen as more "sensual" and "fluid."[25] Yet, these women's writings offer us a contrasting glimpse of the colonial life, which was usually described in writing by men and from a male perspective.[26]

Women who traveled then emerged as a symbol for freedom.[27] Travel increasingly became a part of the modern culture, within which the figure of the tourist, often employing a "Eurocentric gaze," emerged.[28] A more recent and gendered figure in travel is called the "global chick."[29] This figure, although touted as an "ethical model for transnational travel" for being "culturally sensitive" and "accepting of cultural, national, and religious diversity," nonetheless reflects the dominant neoliberal feminism and "hegemonic white feminism" in travel discourses.[30]

To counter this white and neoliberal feminist narrative of the self being responsible for its own happiness and healing, I purposefully tell stories/theories that connect and contextualize my woman-of-color self within the structural/social/political ecologies. By doing so, I am able to introduce a new way of thinking about self-care, self-love, and self-discovery that is outside of the neoliberal feminist framework (e.g., I use the term "emotional contract" rather than the popular and neoliberal concept of "self-care/love" to talk about well-being in chapter 6). I also evade the pervasive neoliberal feminist thinking evident in contemporary and popular women's travel writing by employing a transnational feminist perspective.

## Transnational Feminism

Transnational feminism is "a way of thinking that allows us to understand women's conditions in different locales who nonetheless share similar concerns, the different power relationships among people across and within nations, and the ways in which capitalism, racism, hetero/sexism, and other oppressive systems work in maintaining this unequal power structure across nations."[31] As a perspective, it is often used to discuss issues of migration, diaspora, neocolonialism, "cross-border circulation of people, capital, or ideas," "identity categories [constructed] in historically specific, non-universalizing ways," the "irrelevance of the nation-state in the current phase of globalization," and how "capital and migration" shape "local problems."[32]

In this book, I want to expand the usefulness of transnational feminism to help us think about the gendered and racialized self, particularly in the context of autoethnography and its relationship to affects in the body (rather than the political-economic context), such as pain, as it travels across national borders. By way of a transnational feminist perspective, I frame individual transnational travel as something that can shift one's relationship to pain—and pain here is considered as a node through which power circulates and operates—and can challenge and make visible, rather than reiterate, power structures. The power dynamic I highlight in this book, since I focus on my own travel and pain, consequently revolves around how the "self" is able to negotiate, navigate, and even reclaim power (particularly in relation to pain). My analysis is inevitably registered at an individual level. However, as I hope is evident throughout the chapters, I do not frame the individual as a neoliberal self(ie) who considers healing solely as a personal responsibility.[33] Rather, this book contextualizes the self within the larger (patriarchal/

transnational) structure—personal transformation is always embedded in and demands cultural transformation.

Thus, my position as a woman of color who was born and raised in a third world country and now resides in the United States complicates and repositions the "I" of the traveler's subjectivity. Whereas dominant travel writings often overlook women of color, or represent us as the ones being observed, this book speaks back to these travel writings by projecting the narrative voice of a woman of color in a transnational context.[34]

Because the traveling, moving, and migrating experiences of women of color are significantly different from those of the normative white and/or male body,[35] there can never be a transnational feminist analysis without incorporating women of color's experiences and theories. Throughout the book, I return again and again to the powerful words of Gloria Anzaldúa, Audre Lorde, Inderpal Grewal, Maria Lugones, Sara Ahmed, Devika Chawla, and other feminist theorists of color to help me make sense of what happens.

I also find a transnational feminist perspective helpful in moving us beyond the binary of forced migration versus voluntary travels. As travel bears not only leisure but also nonleisure connotations, such as "expatriation, exile, homelessness, and immigration,"[36] it is important, as transnational feminist scholar Caren Kaplan cautions us, that we move beyond the binary of exile versus pleasure/tourism that operates under the Eurocentric system of representation.[37] What is more important is to understand how power flows transnationally, and how power structures this transnational flow.

I employ a transnational feminist perspective to make visible how, as we travel, we may inevitably support, rather than challenge, capitalism and neoliberalism.[38] The use of the neoliberal apparatus of digital media such as Airbnb, Uber, etc., during my travels, for instance, signals my complicity with the neoliberal and capitalistic power structure. When I attend healing retreats, I contribute to a neoliberal economy that is packaged mostly for middle- and upper-class (often white) people who can afford to carve out unobstructed time to invest in ourselves. These retreats are usually marketed to foreign tourists rather than local residents, and take place in countries where tourism is a continuation of colonial history that perpetuates global inequality, imperialism, and capitalism. In this way, a transnational feminist perspective thus inescapably exposes the class-nation status of the traveler, and how the very act of traveling perpetuates this class-nation structure. As feminist theorist M. Jacqui Alexander argues, "Empire makes all innocence impossible."[39]

I thus write moments of rupture and disjuncture, tension and contention, into the story, rather than erase them in the elusive search for a coherent and innocent narrative. (Throughout the book, the readers will encounter "moments of digression"—where I digress to explain the unequal power relationship present during my travels, which disrupts the otherwise nice flow of the paragraph. I would rather have these moments of digression appear in my book than to privilege the coherence of the story and be complicit in concealing power hierarchy.) I thus invite the readers of this book to keep this in mind while engaging with my stories critically.

To consider travel from a transnational feminist perspective is to understand how travel can be oppressive for marginalized people whose movements are restricted or who do not have the power and privilege to travel due to their lack of "economic wealth and political capital."[40] This means that as I adopt a transnational feminist perspective, I must acknowledge and make visible my privileges, which come, first, from being a tenured associate professor who was on a sabbatical leave (which allowed me the time off from teaching, while still receiving 50 percent of my regular salary) that enabled my year of travel. It is true that, without my sabbatical, I simply could not have afforded such an extended travel—the first ever in my forty years of life. In fact, whenever someone asked me, "How can you afford to travel for a year?" that was my answer: I was on sabbatical, the first one I ever took, ten years after receiving my PhD.

Allow me to digress here, if only to expand on the "How can you afford it?" question that I got asked *a lot*. Some people who asked me this question wanted to know the answer because they dreamed of traveling extensively, too. I am thus sharing my longer answer here, detailing how being on sabbatical works exactly and how I managed the logistics during my year of travel.

There are three pieces of the spending puzzle when I am traveling. First, the food. Receiving guaranteed income during sabbatical meant that I was able to cover my meals no matter where I was. Rather than spending my money to buy food at home in Hawai'i, I would spend it at a market in whatever country I was visiting, where food oftentimes ended up costing less. And when I stayed for more than a week in one place, I would book a place where I could cook. Eating out, just as in Hawai'i, only happened occasionally.

Second, the accommodation. I was able to cover some costs through fellowships and grants, such as a writing fellowship in Catalonia, with room and half-board paid for, or a workshop in Japan with all expenses paid for by the grant our research group received. When my grants or fellowship did not cover my stay, I would tap into the perks of being a part of a diasporic family: having a sister who lives in Canada, a brother in Germany, an uncle in Australia, and parents in Indonesia. My family generously opened their homes for me, as I did for them when they visited me in Hawai'i. These are the places I stayed the longest. At other times, I would rely mostly on relatively inexpensive AirBnB rooms/motels/hostels such as the one I stayed in in Bali for eight dollars a night, or the one in Budapest, which cost twenty-six dollars a night. Booking places sight unseen always carries a risk, of course. Although I often chose a place on the basis of other people's reviews (e.g., on booking.com, I used the filter review score of 8+ and read all their one-star or bad reviews to gauge what the place was like), it did not always work out. The room in Bali for eight dollars a night had a review score of 9, but it had a bathroom so dirty (shall I spare you the shitty details here?—pun slightly intended), I literally did not take a shower or go inside it during my visit, and went to some restaurants' toilets instead. I left the next day. In New Zealand, I was staying at a hostel in a tiny room with two bunk beds with three other strangers. One of them was sick and kept coughing all night. It was before COVID time, but still, I was worried for him (and myself). Most of the times, though, the reviews (and word of mouth from people I knew) kept me from being disappointed or mercilessly scammed. (I went to another cheap place in Bali and had no problems.)

Third, the transportation and tour expenses. Organized tours are usually more expensive than arranging the sightseeing ourselves. Unless it was necessary (e.g., in Iceland, staying at a transparent igloo can only be experienced as part of a tour) or more affordable (e.g., being on a tour boat is cheaper than renting your own private boat!), I always scheduled my own sightseeing. I read reviews and tips on where to go and how to get there, and whenever possible, I would walk or take buses or other affordable means of public transportation. I made sure I had a data plan so I could figure out where I was in case I got lost. (I had a phone plan that included unlimited data in most of the countries I visited, so it did not cost me extra money.) To avoid being stranded in a place where there was no Internet connection, before embarking I would download a map or take pictures of what buses I needed to take. When I needed to fly to my next destination, I relied on Skyscanner to find me some affordable flights (see chapter 1). Being on sabbatical, I was able to be flexible and travel on whatever day and to whatever location was cheapest. A flight from Keflavík International (KEF), Iceland, to Baltimore Washington International (BWI), United States, cost me $189—what a steal, indeed. Thus, for me, being on sabbatical truly afforded me the time and money to travel for a year.

If it seems that I navigated world traveling with relative ease, that is the case because I have yet another privilege in my knapsack: I grew up in an upper-middle-class family in Indonesia who took me traveling often, and by way of doing that, taught me how to travel efficiently. Traveling abroad was not something new for me. I was seven months old when my family first took me to Australia. I was thirteen years old when my parents sent me and my siblings off to stay with our family friend in Japan for a month. When I was sixteen years old, my brother and I visited my sister, who was studying in France at the time. By the time I was nineteen years old, I was traveling to the United States alone for a month, exploring various cities, at times arriving at an airport without already having booked a hotel (the wild times!).

Then, there were privileges that came from being a newly naturalized American citizen. That status freed me from having to worry about acquiring a visa for every country I visited. When I needed a visa, the process was reasonably effortless and efficient. More still, my privilege also came from being able to pass as a heterosexual woman (especially when my white male partner—let us call him Renzo, not his real name—joined me in a few countries), even though I identify as bisexual/wikisexual.[41] My relatively abled and middle-aged body also made travel easier for me than if I had to worry about the still-limited choices of accessible accommodations and sightseeing places across the globe.

To be clear, if I make my privileges visible, I do so not because I want to excuse or recuse myself from them.[42] Instead, I want to remind the readers that these privileges shaped my traveling, thinking, and writing. I want the readers to therefore be suspicious of my stories and me—the "I" or the self in this book (even as I employ a transnational feminist perspective to interrogate power relations) projects an "unreliable narrator voice" nonetheless.[43] I propose here that the knowledge produced in this book resides not only in the theories/stories that I write (or within the book itself) but also in the moments when the readers see what I cannot see for myself because of how my privilege limits the way I view the world. Having privileges can actually be a perspective flaw. Privileges often make us ignorant.

Transnational Feminist Autoethnography: The Personal
Is Epistemological

Autoethnography is a research method that "seeks to describe and systematically analyse (graphy) personal experience (auto) in order to
understand cultural experience (ethno)."[44] The term itself entered the
social sciences world in the 1970s and began to be employed as a more
common method in the 1990s, during a "critical turn in ethnographic
research."[45] Autoethnography is useful when we want to do "something
different with theory and its relation to experience."[46] This method is
particularly apt for me as I aim to use reflexivity and incorporate "intellectual and methodological rigor, emotion, and creativity" to achieve
"social justice and to make life better," which are the core practices of
autoethnography.[47] In employing this method, researchers use their own
experiences as primary data and turn themselves into "experimental
subjects."[48]

By shifting the focus of my research onto myself, autoethnography
allows me to "challenge what counts as data."[49] These personal accounts
are what autoethnographers base their authority on.[50] They contextualize these personal accounts within larger institutional structures that
would then allow them to challenge social inequalities.[51] Clough says
it best when she points out how autoethnography "turn[s] the eye of
the sociological imagination back on the ethnographer" and in this way
reconfigures the existing process of knowledge production.[52]

For me, using transnational feminist autoethnography means turning to my travel journal that I carefully kept throughout the year as my
data. I critically and self-reflectively analyzed these self-as-field notes. I
paid particular attention to my feelings (especially of pain) as an Asian
and transnational scholar who studies transnationalism, race, gender,
and affect/emotion. I also closely contemplated the various techniques
that I used in processing my pain during my travels. I thought about
how transnationalism became the context within which my thoughts
emerged, which then framed the arguments in this book.

To employ a transnational feminist autoethnography is to examine our experiences of traveling/moving across nations, contextualize our research within a transnational context,[53] and draw from transnational feminist theories in producing our knowledge. Such research therefore considers traveling/moving transnationally as essential to the theory that it produces, without which such theory production would not be possible. Transnational feminist autoethnography must therefore incorporate transnational contents, contexts, and processes.

Some of the guiding questions in doing transnational feminist autoethnography are these: *How does movement of human and nonhuman beings, objects, finances, ideas, and/or ideologies affect my lived and intimate experiences, and how I experience my life differently? How does my movement across national boundaries matter in how I experience life and produce knowledge? How do I make connections and comparisons between the different cultures and structures of power (and how they shape the contour and content of my life) encountered during my transnational travels? How do I negotiate and challenge such transnational power as I move across these transnational spaces? What does this transnational movement make possible and visible? How does my self-reflecting on my transnational experiences help contribute to new understandings about something? What transnational cultural practices do I make visible, examine, or criticize by employing transnational feminist autoethnography? How does my form of livability relate to others' in this transnational context? How does what I write help move us toward a feminist future/social justice?* Of course, a transnational feminist autoethnographic work need not address all of these questions or be limited by them. I list them here as a starting point to help us imagine the kinds of questions that may inform transnational feminist autoethnographic research.

In developing transnational feminist autoethnography, I intentionally expand and extend the scholarship of, by, and about women (and marginalized people) of color. This scholarship calls for an autoethnography that centers on women of color, focuses on everyday life and the notion of the personal as political, and is interested in personal transformation as a site of cultural transformation.[54] This means that rather than focusing on big-life-transformation or death/illness narratives, which count as the most dominant story in autoethnographic writings, I make the ordinary of everyday life and "minuscule" transformation the center of my attention.[55]

Transnational feminist autoethnography is also indebted to women of color thinkers in their challenging the traditional autoethnography's "limited notions of the self."[56] They reframe the apolitical "I" (that exists in more traditional autoethnography) to now represent a sociocultural and more political "I." I then use this reframing of the political "I" to rearticulate pain that was previously framed as nonstructural/apolitical (in more traditional autoethnography) as sociocultural and political—not just personal.

Thus, privileging the eye and the emotions of the narrator/traveler self in my stories is done to provide us with a different way to understand ourselves and the structural and the sociopolitical.[57] How the self perceives and tells its story is revealing of the larger structures that allow that story to be told in a particular way from a certain individual perspective. To tell a story is ultimately to locate oneself in history and relations of power.

When locating the self within its larger structural contexts, we must do so *without* the intention to generalize such an experience to a larger group of people.[58] Even the self itself should be constructed not as something that is coherent but rather as something that represents "splitting, conflicting and plural understandings of the self."[59] It is the self that exists at the point of "disjunction"—that is, "between the 'I' who writes and the 'I' who is written about"—and is the site at which "these two selves continually negotiate between themselves."[60] I thus use the self in this book as a point of clarification for theoretical lucidity rather than a point of generalization.

Lastly, I write "the self" as a figure that refers not solely to the author but also to a figurative character that implies and invites into its construction the self of the reader. Doing so allows me to cultivate "a reading voice . . . that constructs the story with [and as] the author," whereby the reader and the author both get to own the story(ies).[61] In other words, the figure of the self becomes a space where the readers can do the work of self-reflection in processing and theorizing how to do things with their own pain.

## Writing Genre in Transnational Feminist Autoethnography

As a last conversation in this chapter on research method, I want us to carefully think about the form or the writing genre. What does a transnational feminist autoethnography work look like? My short answer is, it would look exactly how the author imagines it to be. Preferably, although not necessarily, it would challenge the writing convention in academia.

Let us begin with the norm: autoethnography often leads with stories or uses story as its form of theorizing. In this book, I want to expand the form and genre of autoethnography by using not only stories but also traditional academic theories. At times, I even lead with theory. Theory is part of the story I want to tell. In this way, I want to cling to theory because I dare to stubbornly claim a space and exist in the world of theories where women of color have not always been seriously acknowledged as theorists.

The form that this book takes is indeed different from most autoethnographic works in the field. For instance, Ellis's influential work *Final Negotiations: A Story of Love, Loss, and Chronic Illness* relies more heavily on "story as theory."[62] Her writing is indeed important as it has carved a path for me to produce the kind of writing that uses emotions, stories, and academic theories to make sense of my travels, my life, and my pain—the "evocative autoethnography."[63] However, rather than theorizing mostly through stories, the way that Ellis brilliantly does in her book, I want to chart my own path. I experiment with mixing and merging stories with theories, while allowing each to maintain its shape when it demands it.[64] I let each poke around at the other's boundary.

In combining and critically writing stories and theories as porous, playful, and healing, I evoke Anzaldúa's notion of "autohistoria-teoría," understood as "exceed[ing] the status quo and tak[ing] risks: it combines self-writing with theorizing, fact with fiction, embodiment with knowledge production, and the personal with the social. Key traits include strategic use of fictional, poetic elements; creation of individual/collective selfhoods; use of nonlinear narrative; and acceptance of multiplicity-multiple realities, truths, perspectives, epistemologies, and worlds."[65] The spirit of Anzaldua's "autohistoria-teoría" indeed perfectly captures, as well as haunts and grounds, my writing.[66]

I offer the stories in this book as *my* interpretation of what happened, my way of putting words around the perception of pain in a legible order (while simultaneously questioning that very technology of legibility). I consider stories as "creations, not discoveries of absolute truths," as they "re-scribe and re-tell," rather than "describe the world."[67] The relationship between story and truth is always fraught, even in those stories claiming to be nonfiction. My story is thus meant to probe and proximate (rather than claim) the truths of pain. Story is but a way to represent what is perceived to be the form that truth and reality take.[68] This is how I approach autoethnography, storytelling, and academic writing in this book.

Last but not least, I want to make explicit my intention to write in the form that challenges the normative convention of autoethnographic and academic writing. First, I do so because I want to answer the call from communication studies scholar Devika Chawla, who courageously asks us to disinherit the writing skills we learned in academia, which work to keep us apolitical, and our knowledge harmless to the status quo.[69] My book does not fit in familiar genres of travel writing (because this book is *not* a book *about* travel—it is about pain) or academic text (because this book incorporates memoir—thereby pushing the boundaries of an academic text—and structures its thoughts in ways that may not be familiar to academic readers). There is a chapter that focuses intensely on theory, another on story, and yet another one on the structural contexts of specific countries. They do not follow a formula. They may not always resemble one another. There is no pattern in how I write these chapters.

I recognize, however, that by writing in a form that does not fit neatly in existing genres (e.g., autoethnographic, autobiographical, or academic writing), I may disorient the readers.[70] But hopefully, I can then reorient the readers to something else, to a different way of engaging with the world and the thoughts circulating in it. Thus, I consider creating disorientation and disruption in the text as necessary and crucial, if we are to create a rupture in how we understand and have a more transgressive relationship with knowledge and how it is produced and consumed.[71]

Second, I write in the form that I hope will be more inviting for general readers because I want the book itself to do the work of bridging and healing the distrust between academics and the public. There is too much pain in this world already. I want to offer this book as that which can hopefully soften the suffering, rather than deepen the divide.

3

## How Can I Perceive Differently?

I grew up hearing stories of my father's infidelity. Why people would tell me those stories, I do not know. What I do know is that I have stitched his stories with my own. I weave his endless betrayals with those of the different lovers in my life, and learn that love burns and breaks more than just the heart. Throughout the years, I have learned that it is not safe to love. But how are we to learn to access love when a love relationship was passed down as something painful?

There I was, on the road in Costa Rica. My partner, Renzo, was driving. We had been exploring the country, staying at a treehouse in Monteverde, spotting a tarantula during a guided jungle night tour in Manuel Antonio, and watching sunset at an estuary beach while eating ribeye steak served on a preheated volcanic rock, and sipping some Carambola Colada in Tamarindo. So far so delicious.

But the main reason we were in Costa Rica at all was that Renzo had been wanting to visit this one particular yoga retreat center. We were sort of saving it, expecting it to be the best, for last. And that is where we were driving to that late afternoon. The resort was located in Nosara, the Guanacaste province, about a two-hour drive from Tamarindo, where we had stayed the night before. At the resort, we had hoped to take random yoga classes and surfing lessons on some days, and be intentionally slothful on other days.

But that was before Renzo blurted out an innocent but perky, "Oh, I know her!"—and that changed everything.

Those were definitely not the words I had expected him to say when I read him an announcement from the retreat center's website: that there was a women-only healing retreat that started that night, and one of the retreat facilitators/yoga teachers who was living in Costa Rica at the time actually came from the same city as he did.

Suddenly, I felt a gnawing tug in my stomach. *Did he persist on paying the extra money for this overpriced retreat center because he was smitten by the yoga teacher?* I remembered him mentioning her name when she was guest teaching at the yoga studio he always went to, and that he liked her. But I did not think that he would fly across the globe just to see her again. It then made sense to me why he was so persistent in choosing that exact resort, even when I had tried to convince him to book another place that was much cheaper and just as nice.

When I asked him about it, he assured me that he did not like her in that way. He liked her teaching style, he told me. His tone was even light and airy, with a hint of warm sweetness, like that first bite of freshly made lemon meringue. It annoyed me that he could be that cheery in the midst of a brewing drama. *How could people be that happy all the time?* Sometimes I wondered what could burst his bubbly way of being. Even when two of his close friends died, he did not cry. *Is that how we are supposed to feel when we do yoga every day? Maybe I should do yoga more often.*

Whatever the intensity, degree, or category of "like" he felt for her, I figured he must have liked her enough to travel the world and spend some extra money to stay at a place where he knew she would be teaching yoga. If this had been an isolated incident, I would have found his "alleged" crush to be somewhat cute, adorable even. But this happened after my finding out (more like snooping around his text messages) that he had been having coffees, lunches, and wine with a few other women, and had lied about it.

## My Impromptu Retreat

As soon as we checked into our room, I emailed the retreat leader and inquired whether I could join her program even though I had missed their first day, which was the night I arrived. She responded right away and welcomed me to her eight-day retreat—unfortunately, I had to also miss the last day. I told Renzo of my changed plans; he stuck to his plans of taking surfing and yoga classes. (I must admit that this was one of the things I appreciated about Renzo: rarely, if ever, did he complain about my [change of] plans, even when he did not end up being included in them. Another piece of evidence that nothing seemed to easily burst his happy bubble.)

I showed up the next morning to a group of twelve women, including the retreat facilitator, who had gone through the first ice-breaker experience the previous night. We were going around the room, sharing stories of pain that we had been carrying in our lives. But as I was sitting in the circle listening to the group talk, I felt at home right away. I was fluent in the language of pain and sadness. I can even say it is my mother tongue. I had learned it since birth. Even when I joined the retreat late, I was able to catch up with the group's conversation without any problems.

The retreat's program had a set daily schedule that began with morning yoga and meditation, followed by breakfast and the first workshop session. Lunch marked the midpoint of the day. (For lunch and dinner, I usually joined Renzo at locally owned restaurants where "locals" went to eat. We wanted to avoid playing the role of the "ugly tourists." But I realize now that this desire only made us uglier: Who are we to invade the local hangouts with our bodies, taking up spaces so that people living there would now have to wait in line just to get lunch? Increased popularity among tourists also means that these places that were once affordable for locals became more expensive. We are not "savvy travelers" for going where the locals go. We are ignorant invaders.) Lunch was then followed by a couple of hours of free time. Most participants usually used this time to lounge around the infinity pool, surrounded by the luscious greenery of the Costa Rican jungle. Afternoon yoga preceded watching the sunset and dinner. Finally, a second workshop at night sealed the daily schedule.

Of all the retreat participants in our group, only one woman came from the local community. This is not unlike most other retreats I have been to, where most participants come from Western countries. The retreat fee might explain the why of that. The minimum wage in Costa Rica is between 286,000 and 615,000 Colón per month, or 460–985 USD;[1] most retreats charge more than 2,000 USD a week, making it harder for most local people to participate. Except for the one woman from Costa Rica, the rest of the participants came from the United States—they were mostly the facilitator's yoga students. Because of this, the retreat language was English. Only three women, including myself, were nonwhite. It is worthy of note that the retreat center was owned by a North American family.[2] To provide a context, out of more than five million people in Costa Rica, about 120,000 Americans live there, and about 1.4 million Americans visit the country every year, making the United States the main source of tourism in Costa Rica.[3]

During the retreat, the facilitator had the participants share stories and do activities that would transform our pain, and turn us into healed and happy women.[4] For this impromptu retreat, I inevitably worked on trust and infidelity issues—what with Renzo's hot yoga teacher crush and other lies. These issues are the thorns that make palpable the places of pain in my relationship(s), provide the context and container for the pain I have been carrying that connected my father's love stories to my own, and, most importantly for this chapter, function as a site for my theorizing pain and perception.

Thus, I will first share the story that I was working on at the retreat. Then, I will use it to explain the different and problematic ways we have been taught to perceive, and explore what it means to perceive differently. What would happen if I had perceived Renzo's response, "Oh, I know her!" differently? Would I then not have felt the silent but raging pain as strongly as I did? That is indeed the point that I would like to explore and explain in this chapter: when we shift how we perceive, we will have a different relationship with pain.

To be clear, what I am advocating is *not* a simple shift in perception, from a negative-thinking "I" to a positive-thinking "I." The "I" I am referring to here is an "I" within the context of its society. This means that the question of how I perceive is also a question that implores us to ask, What does our society teach us about how to perceive? Is our perception "docile"? Does it make us docile? Does it create more pain in our lives? If it does, how can we perceive in ways that do not provoke even more pain and that liberate us from the shackles of societal gendered norms? In other words, how can we perceive differently?

## The Story: The Love of My Father's Life

If my father were ever capable of loving someone, she might just be the love of his life. Let us call her Shinta (not her real name). She has been my father's mistress for thirty-three years. How they can stay together for over three decades is a mystery to me. During the decades of my father's marriage to my mother, he has not only had Shinta as a mistress but he also has had more than a dozen affairs, and a religious marriage that did not last long to a B-list celebrity. (In Indonesia, Moslems are allowed to have four wives.) But Shinta has been the only one he has "kept" for decades, besides my mother, until today. From what my father told me, he sort of fell in love with her as he was stepping in to help take care of her family financially—she is part of our extended family. Yes, my father's mistress, the love of his life, is a close family relative.

My father was a tall, charming, and handsome (but not necessarily humble) man. He often bragged about how good-looking he was—he often attributed this to his mixed ancestry of Arab, Chinese, and Javanese people. He was always the life of the party, telling one dirty joke after another. He was the kind of person who would randomly approach strangers, including foreign tourists, spouting whatever words he knew in the language of the tourist he was talking to, and make them laugh.

Although Shinta is part of our extended family, I cannot remember much about her. I cannot even recall ever having had an actual conversation with her during any of the family gatherings, if she ever came at all. *How does she feel about her relationship with my father? Does she truly love him? Does she ever get jealous of my mother? What burns deep within her?* I wish I could ask her these questions and get to know her better as a person, a woman. But growing up, our parents forbade us from contacting her or her family, although they never told us why. (I recognize, of course, that she might not even want to know me/us either.) Nonetheless, and unbeknownst to her, Shinta was my life-defining moment. She turned me into the kind of person that I became in my romantic relationships.

It was late afternoon. I was perhaps nineteen years old, and my brother, fourteen. My brother was just like any other teenager who liked to watch porn. He especially liked going through my father's secret collections because it was fun to find tapes in different hiding places. It was like a scavenger hunt. But for porn videos. And he was really good at it, too. He always managed to find one or more of those Betamax videos somewhere around the house. Jakarta, the capital of Indonesia, in the mid-1990s was just beginning to transition from Betamax to LaserDisc. But these pirated porn videos that my brother watched at home were mostly in Betamax.

That afternoon was no different. He was home alone. Sort of. As in most other upper-middle-class homes in Jakarta at the time, the domestic helpers and family driver also lived with us, but they hung out in the back of the house. Wanting to watch some porn, my brother looked around the house and found none. But when he went through our father's briefcase, he found two and watched them both. Quietly.

"Do you want to watch Dad's sex videos? Like with Dad in it?" I remember him asking me as soon as I got home from campus that afternoon. His tone was cool and calm. Like he was just pointing out the color of his jacket or the sky. Blue. Not light blue. Not pastel blue. Not baby blue. Just blue. No particular emotion there.

*What? What did he say?* I wasn't sure if I had heard him correctly. But if he had said what I thought he had said, would I want to see it? I cringed.

I sat down next to my brother on the couch.

"You ready?" he asked and pressed the play button.

There were a man and a woman in the missionary position, shot from behind. You could not really tell who was who. But when the man rolled over to the side and tried to fix the camera, I could see him, my father, in his nakedness. I tried not to see his penis.

"They're not doing some crazy techniques here. Is Mom really that bad in bed? I don't know why people keep saying that it's because she didn't know how to serve him in bed that he keeps cheating on her. But there you go, you better know how to be good in bed if you want to keep your man." His comment was innocent—as innocent as a fourteen-year-old boy who watched his father's sex tape could be. But his comment was one that I had heard too often: if you want to keep your man, you better know how to keep his penis happy. Even popular transnational women's magazines such as *Cosmopolitan*, including *Cosmopolitan Indonesia*, make a lot of money off this premise. (I suppose femininity and sexuality are never only locally, but also transnationally, constructed.)

My brother did not play the whole video. He ejected the first one and inserted the second one. The video player made a gentle buzzing sound as it swallowed the video inside its body.

"This one is where she fucked Dad's friend."

I sat there, not knowing what to think. Perhaps thinking was unnecessary. The sex tape had already found its way into my subconscious mind, rearranging my desire-map, and redirecting the course of my own sexual development. I did not realize how something that seemed so trivial could become so pivotal in my life, until the trauma of that moment shaped (or scarred) how I relate romantically with others.

Years after, that is, after many, many failed romantic relationships, I realized that seeking my father's love, I must have turned myself into Shinta—at least, the part of her that I thought my father must have fallen in love with. The Shinta in the Sex Tape. The Shinta with her sexual magic.[5] In my attempts to be like her—the one who became the love of my father's life—I turned myself into a woman who was obsessed with mastering new sexual techniques. I took all kinds of sex-related workshops (from how to best give a hand job, a blow job, or any kind of job there is, really, to how to safely practice BDSM to how to breathe my way into blissful orgasm the Tantra way). I was also addicted to buying sexy lingerie—perhaps I was trying to cover up what was lacking on the inside (i.e., sexual confidence) with something pretty on the outside. Yet, none of these "tricks" helped me with my romantic relationships. At least, the part where they were supposed to make me the love of their life.

And there I was, at a women's healing retreat in Costa Rica, finding out that the main reason Renzo chose that specific retreat center was that he was smitten by his white, young, twenty-something, beautiful, and incredibly sexy yoga instructor. She had the kind of magnetic beauty and delicate sensuality that pulled you in. A woman whom I secretly, too, found incredibly attractive, and wanted for myself. How ironic.

## Pain and Perception

The first big question in this book is, How can I perceive differently? It matters that we ask this question because how we perceive ultimately contributes to whether or not we experience an event as painful. Do we perceive in ways that the dominant power structure tells us to and that often contribute to more pain, or do we defy it?

The mantra that I want the readers to remember is this: *pain does not exist outside of perception.* This is not the same as saying that the pain is only in your mind or, worse, that you need to just "suck it up"—this would be horrible and hurtful to the person hearing it. First of all, remember that pain is not the actual tumor or blister itself. Second, this book acknowledges that pain *is* the way of (a feminist) life. It is here to stay, and it is part of our bodily living (but "exterior" or external to the body—remember the hermit crab shell metaphor in chapter 1 here). Because it is part of our life, we might as well figure out a better way to carry it. One way that this book proposes that we do that is to critically, creatively, and differently engage with our perception.

Perception is key in understanding and carrying pain because pain is but an integrated and intricate process of *perceiving* the wound through various modalities—pain is not merely a bodily sensation.[6] Perception also matters because we often consider it to be an "access to the truth" and a means of knowing and making sense of the world/wound. In other words, it helps us register whether or not the wound/event is painful, how intense the pain is, and how to relate to it.[7]

If perception sits at the center of pain experience, then, should we not be questioning and unpacking it when we want to better carry or understand pain? Absolutely. It is this relationship between perception and pain that I want us to mull over more carefully in the second part of this chapter. I want to follow the logic that if perception shapes the experience of pain, then that experience will inevitably change when we shift our perception and our understanding of perception.

We need to unpack the relationship between pain and perception because power operates through the controlling mechanism of pain. A way of perceiving that hurts us works to control and discipline us. To carry pain differently, we must unlearn how we have perceived in docile ways, and learn new modes of perceiving.

To explain my point better, I will show first how I perceived during my retreat, then how the disciplinary process of perceiving works, and finally how we can find alternative and more subversive ways to perceive. I use the retreat experience as an example to discuss the relationship between pain and perception because it was there where I was able to make the connections between how one is *trained* to perceive, how perception is used to discipline and make us docile and support the dominant ideology, and how this docile perception may cause us pain. Thus, by using the retreat as an example for this chapter, I hope it will become easier and clearer for the readers to follow my point. Lastly, the retreat also works as a perfect site of analysis because healing retreats often function as spaces where we flex and make flexible our pain.

Of course, the process of learning how to perceive does not only happen at these healing retreats. The disciplining process of perceiving happens every day through conversations we have with friends, families, and coworkers. We also learn how to perceive when we watch movies, interact on social media, and however else we engage with the outside world.

At a methodological level, I focus on the retreat as it reflects my transnational feminist autoethnography method. Had I not traveled to that specific retreat in Costa Rica, and found out about Renzo's crush, gone through the retreat's activities and programs, and reflected on them through a feminist lens and through the perspective of pain as an anamorphic apparatus, I would not have come up with the knowledge/theory for this chapter. That is, it is in the act of *crossing* these national boundaries that knowledge is produced.

## In the Beginning, There Was Arrogant Perception

In spending almost a week with these strong, brave, and inspiring women, being a witness to their (and my own) pain and how we all transform that pain, I noticed the carefully choreographed ways in which we move from a victim to a victor subjectivity.

In the beginning, all retreat participants were asked to dive, heart first, into our (childhood) trauma. Everyone, without exception, shared stories that positioned them as the noble victim and the perpetrator as evil. In the story about my father, I positioned myself as an innocent victim of child abandonment and emotional abuse. I portrayed my father as the absent father, an evil patriarch who oppressed my mother and had extramarital affairs with several women, including the one with a close family relative. Through his manipulation and control (not to mention the belt-whip on our backs, which was a common practice then, to make us succumb to his power), he managed to silence us.

Critically reflecting back on this, I notice that everyone's story (mine included) followed a script that law professor Isabelle Gunning calls an "arrogant perception." Arrogant perception is a perception that "sees himself [*sic*] as the center of the universe."[8] Through this lens, we see ourselves as better than the other (in this case, the perpetrator), who is perceived "as a lesser or defective form of the self."[9] We become the "noble" victims and coherent subjects who are morally superior to the perpetrators. We see perpetrators as the bad actors and *only* bad, without fully contextualizing their lives and actions in the historical, political, etc., structure that makes it possible for them to act in such a way to begin with. The perpetrator does not even have their own independent perceptions, except for those we "impose" on them.[10]

When we see from an arrogant perspective, we tend to "falsif[y] and oversimplif[y]."[11] For instance, I oversimplified who my father was by omitting stories of the times he paid attention to us as a family, took us on family vacations, instilled in us a love for traveling and paid for our world travels, treated our family to nice restaurants or cooked us delicious meals, or gave me advice when I ran my own small businesses in Indonesia. There were moments of his generosity that did not appear in my story.

In projecting arrogant perception, I failed to see that both the perpetrator and the victim are "victims" of patriarchy. This means that patriarchy produces subjects who do things the way that they do. (I invoke the word "patriarchy" as a concept that is intersectional—not only gendered but also racialized, hetero/sexualized, capitalist, imperialist, and so on.) For instance, in Indonesia it is quite common, even encouraged, that men with means have mistresses. It signifies their masculinity and class status.

When I processed what happened through my arrogant perception, I felt a sense of overwhelming pain, hopelessness, and insignificance, even as I claimed the nobler standpoint. Although it may feel good for me to claim that someone else did something wrong and to even claim that my trust issues in romantic relationships stem from my father's infidelity, arrogant perception does nothing to change my life or his, let alone break patriarchy. This way of perceiving keeps me in my victimhood, my docile position.

Arrogant perception even sets me up for further heartbreak and emotional pain because through this lens, I am stuck in the blaming game that continues to overemphasize my father's role in directing the trajectory of my life. By perceiving that my father, my partner, and men in general cannot be trusted, I am also complicit in perpetuating the idea that they are not multidimensional beings living in a complex and intersectional power hierarchy.

This is not to suggest that I condone their behavior or that I blame myself for feeling what I feel. Rather, I am pointing out that when I perceive through an arrogant eye, through the way I have learned to perceive, which follows a dominant cultural script, I am not able to see beyond the limitation of my own perception. Arrogant perception is indeed limiting and limited. It justifies our pain but does not encourage us to transcend it or to challenge the patriarchal structure that creates the conditions for people to act in hurtful ways in the first place.

### Then, There Was Loving Perception

After asking us to share our trauma, the retreat leader then skillfully executed other insightful and thoughtfully planned activities and conversations that helped us deconstruct and rewrite our stories, our past, and our future. To induce a shift in perception and reframe our trauma, the retreat leader provided us with short articles for us to read. Then, we had to respond to the various prompts that she created.[12] We were asked to see our parents or whoever caused us pain from a different perspective that is more compassionate.

This activity reminded me of the concept of the "loving eye" that feminist theorist Marilyn Frye coined, which Gunning argues can function as the antidote to arrogant perception. In seeing through loving perception, we were able to see the perpetrators in their cultural and patriarchal contexts—most of the traumas shared during the retreat originated from gender-specific roles or were a form of gender-based sexual violence.[13] We perceived more compassionately our fathers and all others who wounded us, for we could see how their acts were reflections of the cultures that enabled them to enact such violent or violating behaviors. Their behavior is not a statement about who they/we really are—that there is something wrong with them/us. It is not about us or them per se but about the structure that allows it to happen.

In this way of perceiving, both the victims and the perpetrators are positioned as complex intersectional beings.[14] We understand and become more compassionate not only toward the perpetrators but also toward ourselves in reacting and feeling the way that we did. As an example, to see my father from a loving perception was to reflect back on how in 2016 when I visited him in Jakarta, he asked me to accept his apology for abandoning us and told me that he had stopped seeing Shinta. (Of course, that ended up being another lie.)

The 2016 apology had indeed allowed me to see my father's world through his eyes. I was able to comprehend that he truly did not see anything wrong with what he had done. He really believed that he was "helping" Shinta and her family, and that it is natural for men to have the kind of sexual desire that he had, and to act on it. He even complained to me that it was actually hard to keep two wives (my mother and the B-list celebrity) happy. He told me,

I remember praying to God and asking Him, "If I were meant to have two wives, please give me the strength to be with both of them. If not, please distance me from the young one." He answered my prayer. I grew tired of the young one because she was so possessive. But your mom, she was suffering inside but she always treated me nicely. . . . Did you know? Every afternoon, this was when your [older] sister was three or four years old, your mother would walk me to the door and send me off with a sweet face, and every night, when I came home from the young wife's house after midnight, she would open the door for me and serve me a cup of hot tea. Every night, always like that. But after a while, it was too exhausting for me. Can you imagine? After coming home from work, I had to take a shower, drive all the way to the young wife's house, spend time with her, and then come back home to your mother. Too exhausting.

The audacity to share this story to provoke some sympathy from me (*did he?*) aside, it situates him in his historical context, exposes his beliefs and behaviors as part of his cultural values, and allows me to see the complexity of a man raised in a deeply patriarchal culture. When we see the other's behavior as reflecting the dominant culture that enables and teaches them how to behave, rather than indicating a pure malicious intent to hurt us, we begin to craft a space of compassion for the other/ perpetrator and even for ourselves. Loving perception is indeed more intersectional, mindful, and context conscious than arrogant perception.

However, loving perception, especially toward the oppressor, can still be toxic. Even as I was able to consider my father in a more loving and compassionate light, it did nothing to challenge his power and the patriarchy itself, which were the sources of the problem. Loving perception does not answer the questions of why we perceive the way that we do and what (ideological-emotional) work perceptions do (e.g., how they contribute to the pain we are feeling). We overlook how subjects/ subjectivities and their perceptions are produced and disciplined under dominant discourses and ideologies. We are still docile subjects who are complicit within a dominant way of perceiving others, albeit in a more loving way. Loving perception is, after all, a script, a "trained" perception, a docile perception, and therein lies the problem.

### Yet, There Was Always the Docile Perception

The carefully thought out activities and programs that took place throughout the week helped the retreat participants move from portraying ourselves as victims of abandonment and emotional/sexual/ physical abuse to reclaiming our power, femininity, and bold and bodacious womanhood. At the end of the retreat, the retreat leader asked us to write down any revelations we had experienced and to come up with plans for after the retreat. We were asked to re/envision ourselves anew.

This is what I wrote, scribbling notes on the pages of the retreat workshop book:

"I need to take up space and be loud."

"When triggered, we first need to unhook. Don't take the emotional bait."

"I'm not the one to help [my mother]. . . . She needs to step up and be her own hero."

"Get off the jealousy boat and get on another boat."

"Is this what I am competing against [in reference to the yoga teacher whom Renzo was infatuated with]? I am a kind person and I take really good care of you [Renzo]. If this is not enough, if I am not enough for you, then, forget it. Someone else will worship the ground I walk on."

"This is not the life I want to live. This is not the feeling I want to have in a relationship."

Finally, an excerpted note to myself:

I want you to always remember this: Believe in your own magic. Find Beauty and Love in everything and everyone you encounter. Be generous with your love. You will never run out of it. Remember to step into your Clarity so you can provide wise counsel to yourself and others. Don't feel insecure. Don't ever, ever, ever, ever make anyone else's world small because you don't know how to love them. Remember to always stop and sit and meditate. Remember to always be grateful. Remember to have confidence. Remember your capacity to weave magic into your life. Remember that living and following your intuition and pleasure is the only way to live, the only life worth living. . . .

You have done so much in this life. You have showed up in awe-inspiring ways for yourself and for others who are so lucky to have crossed paths with you. You are strong, courageous, and brave. I admire you. There is nothing in this world that you cannot handle. I trust you. I want you to trust Life.

These notes, where I shared new perceptions of myself, function as evidence that I have transformed my pain and victimhood subjectivity, and that I will live my life fully and affirm my own sense of self without seeking external validation. In writing them, I followed a cultural script that teaches us how to be a "good" victor: someone who has overcome the obstacles in their life (even though in reality I may not know how to actually practice being a strong, courageous, and brave woman in my daily life).

First, I must note that the logic of this personal transformation is neoliberal in that individuals are asked to solve their problems by way of imagining a new and more empowered version of themselves, rather than also being asked to challenge the patriarchal structure (e.g., sexism, rape culture, etc.) that hurts us. The retreat itself operates within and functions to uphold neoliberalism and consumerism. To clarify, I am not singling out the retreat I attended in Costa Rica as neoliberal. Most retreats I have attended are indeed neoliberal, and they follow a similar structure in encouraging personal transformation. They tell us that the pain that we are feeling can be healed if only we can change ourselves (and spend enough money on the right products), or go to retreats and workshops such as these to invest in ourselves. These businesses of (mostly white) Americans hosting retreats in countries that build their economies on Western tourism do indeed capitalize on the self-help economy of neoliberalism and capitalism.

Second, and more directly related to the point I am making in this chapter, these programs and activities function as a site where we are being taught *how* to perceive and are being supervised and disciplined in that training. The retreat teaches us how to create a new "habituated way of perceiving."[15] From arrogant perception that sees myself as the victim to loving perception that compassionately sees the other in their own context to reframing myself as the "strong, courageous, and brave" victor, these perceptions exemplify what I call "docile perception."

I develop the concept of docile perception by drawing from philosopher Michel Foucault's notion of "docile bodies," which he observes as a historically new project emerging in the eighteenth century.[16] For readers who may not be familiar with the concept of docile bodies, perhaps an example could be helpful here. A gendered docile body may look like a woman who sits with her legs closed or crossed, whereas a man may sit with his legs wide open.[17] It is not that women and men inherently want to sit in this way. Rather, it is that growing up, girls are taught and disciplined to sit (or talk, walk, feel, dress, etc.) in this feminine way.

In a nutshell, the notion of docile bodies speaks to the regulation of bodies (when, where, how, and what the body should do) as a form of self-discipline, and as a self-imposed articulation and subjection of power. The docility project thus works at the level of the individual by way of "supervising the processes of the activity rather than its result," and it works through "a subtle coercion."[18]

Building on Foucault's notion of docile bodies, I propose the term "docile perception" to make visible the disciplined ways in which we perceive. Through this concept, I also want to emphasize that it is "the processes of the activity" of perceiving that are constantly being supervised (think here of the retreat functioning as a panopticon).[19] Disciplining the process of perception means that what (i.e., the *object* of perception) and how (i.e., the *process* of perception) we perceive are constantly supervised. Once it is fully internalized, the practice of docile perception is self-imposed and self-regulated at the individual level, and it often works to oppress us and make us docile.

If docility of the body means that "the body was to be trained, exercised, and supervised,"[20] docility of perception means that what is being "trained, exercised, and supervised" is our perception. At the retreat, for instance, when the participants were asked to trace their emotional wound to a particular event or person, we were taught to identify a legible script that would allow others to understand the origin of our pain story, and to abide by such a script in telling our story.

The exercises that asked us to tell a story from a specific point of perception are thus examples of a *process* that disciplines our perception and the narrativity of that perception (i.e., how one tells the story based on how one perceives). For instance, arrogant perception is a form of docile perception because when telling a story through an arrogant eye, I subscribe to the dominant script of what it means to be a "good" victim: someone who is innocent and does not challenge the perpetrator (even though in reality I did). As arrogant perceivers, we focus our stories mostly on the harmful behavior of the other as a result of their choices or character flaws rather than the structure that enables such behavior. In focusing on their behavior, we leave the structure of power unquestioned. We also feel righteous in our pain, and are invested more in our pain than in bringing down the dominant ideology.

When we were then asked to recognize the conditions of possibility within which the harmful behavior of the other is produced—through a loving perception—we were being trained to see from a different perspective. In my case, I learned to shift how I see my father, and to locate him within the patriarchal culture that enabled and encouraged his behavior. Nonetheless, loving perception, as yet another form of docile perception, only changes how we feel toward others/ourselves, but it does not change the structure of power within which these behaviors are enacted as a function of a subjectivity within the dominant discourse. Moreover, the fact that neoliberalism governs this or other self-help retreats, or that the retreat itself is a form of a neoliberal business run by a white American taking mostly white Americans to Costa Rica, also remains unchallenged.

A perception is docile when it supports and does not challenge the dominant ideology. Docile perception makes us docile subjects who do not question how perception works to support the dominant ideology. For instance, patriarchy as the dominant ideology benefits from my ability to lovingly perceive my father as a man who believes that it is his duty to "save" women by marrying them or making them his mistress (so he can uplift these women's living conditions). Because it functions to serve the dominant ideology, docile perception further disempowers and is often injurious to the perceiving (and perceived) subject. It keeps us in our docile and gendered emotional habitus, and works to maintain the status quo. The sexist law that allows a man to have four wives, but a woman to have only one husband, or the gendered economy that privileges men to earn and accumulate more money than women, remains unchallenged. It is these sexist laws and practices that are at the root of the problems that need to be destroyed first, if we are to ever truly and fully address the pain in our lives.

That our perception is being supervised and disciplined means that if we do not follow the script and perceive in the way that we are supposed to, we are seen as a threat to the existence of the group and therefore in need of control.[21] For instance, if at the end of the retreat I do not claim my empowered, whole, and healed status, and proclaim that I am a new woman, free from my emotional pain, I will be pushed and asked further questions to help me get to that point of the new empowered self. There was no space for me to say otherwise. Indeed, each one of the participants, without fail, managed to ascend to their new self. We all have internalized what we are supposed to say and do during these retreats.

When a person is docile, they do "not have to be externally policed,"[22] because they have internalized the values of and are being controlled through dominant "discourses, practices, and institutions" that are circulated and implemented to support these docility projects.[23] Discourses such as feminist or antifeminist discourse, trauma discourse, survivor discourse, spiritual discourse, etc., shape what and how we perceive. They provide us with a script for how to think, feel, and talk about what happens.[24] For example, in trauma discourse, there are scripts that tell us how to feel toward the traumatic event.[25] After experiencing sexual violation, a woman survivor may feel shame rather than anger. The woman may feel that this is what she *really* feels. However, what she may not realize is that her feeling of shame reflects the "culturally conditioned way of perceiving [that] is prior to perception itself."[26] She is following a "script" that has existed prior to the event.[27] To clarify, I am not at all saying that she does not know how or what to feel, or that what she feels is wrong. That would be dismissive of her feeling. What I am saying is that her/our perception/feeling may seem true or natural and normal to her/us because it has been part of her/our culture for decades and, certainly, prior to the moment of perception/feeling itself.

Moreover, when we share how we feel with others, we recirculate the script/discourse and teach others about how to feel/perceive when experiencing sexual abuse. Hence, the fact that we "inherit a set of 'scripts' for how to interpret reality,"[28] and we follow and communicate with others through it, is an example of how discourse works to produce subjects who are docile in our way of perceiving reality.

I also want to make clear here that I do not argue that docile perception causes pain in a direct, simple, and straightforward manner. Rather, I want to point out that when we perceive in docile ways, we perceive as a function of a historically specific subjectivity, entering a historically specific discourse that has existed (and was normalized) long before we entered into such a discourse.

To better explain this point, I want to use an example of the moment when I realized that Renzo's insistence on staying at that specific resort was related to his yoga teacher crush. When I felt jealous (rather than angry at or questioning of patriarchy and monogamy), I followed a dominant script that had existed long prior to the event. My perception is a function of a well-known subjectivity—"a jealous woman/lover"—within the historically specific dominant discourse of monogamous romantic relationship. My docile perception reflects the dominant cultural scripts that prescribe how I should react and behave in a monogamous and committed relationship when presented with the situation: that I should demand that Renzo only desire me and me alone, that I should deem unacceptable his desire for other women, and that I need to feel jealous of the other woman. My perception is docile when I perceive from the subjectivity of an arrogant perceiver who positions myself as the noble victim morally superior to Renzo (as if I have never desired other people—not even Idris Elba?—during our time together). Focusing on the individual's/Renzo's behavior, rather than the structure, I fail to challenge the ageist, sexist, and patriarchal structure that enables and even encourages heterosexual men to fancy much younger women who embody the white beauty standard.

My perception is docile in that it reflects and supports the dominant discourses and historically specific subjectivities that precede and shape my perception. When I perceive in docile ways, from the subjectivity of a jealous woman in a monogamous relationship, I serve the interests of the dominant group that tells us that monogamy is *the only* way to be in a romantic relationship. Remember, monogamy has not always been the dominant mode of romantic relationship throughout times, places, and cultures. Philosopher Friedrich Engels in *The Origin of the Family, Private Property, and the State*, for instance, theorizes that the nuclear (heterosexual) family, a monogamous coupling, is constructed as part of the capitalist system within which men want to be certain that it is their children (and not other men's) who will inherit their property.[29] Feminist Shulamith Firestone in her book *The Dialectic of Sex* has criticized romanticism (also in a heterosexual relationship context) as a dominant ideology, a "cultural tool of male power," that functions to oppress women and subjugate them, and keep them "from knowing their condition" (e.g., by way of exploiting women's labor to take care of the home and the children for free so that men can work outside the home).[30] This means that when I arrived at the point of finding out about Renzo's crush, which provoked my jealousy, the ideology of romantic love and monogamous relationship had already been so naturalized and embedded in the norm of my everyday life that I was not even aware of how they shaped my feelings and perceptions of the event. I forgot that how I behaved (as a jealous lover) reflected and supported this ideology. And that by perceiving in the way that I did (in docile ways), I kept the hegemony of monogamy (and the jealous/lover subjectivity) in its place.[31]

As a last note in this section, I need to explicitly say that in revealing the docile perception that was operating at this retreat, I do not intend to dismiss such a powerful gathering, one that was organized and attended by women, and centered around transforming our pain. Nor do I wish to trivialize the traumatizing events in our pasts or the feelings that all of us experienced during the retreat. Rather, my goal is to illuminate the working of a disciplinary process of perceiving that shows how power operates through how we perceive, which reflects the ever-present and simultaneously invisible dominant power.[32] I hope these healing retreats (and all of us, really) can morph their/our way into becoming sites where we challenge rather than be complicit in the process and project of producing the docility of perception.

## What Is the Alternative? From Docile to Defiant Perception

To change and challenge docile perception, we need more than a shift in perspective. It is not enough, for instance, to shift from an arrogant to a loving perception because both still function as docile perception.[33] If we liken arrogant perception to negative thinking, and loving perception to positive thinking, both of these ways of thinking (and perceiving) are nonetheless problematic (even as positive thinking makes us feel better), because they do not challenge the conditions and structures of power that produce pain in the first place.

Thus, we need a different mode of perceiving. I propose here but one alternative way of perceiving that may move us away from docile perception: I call it "defiant perception"—a perception that rejects, resists, and rebels against the disciplined and dominant ways of perceiving. Cultivating a more rebellious perception is important as it aims to challenge the dominant power structure rather than perpetuate it.

One may wonder, Does it matter whether or not we consider perception as docile or defiant when we can feel the pain nonetheless? I argue that it does matter. By defying and disrupting our normative/disciplined way of perceiving, we can alter our relationship to pain, while changing and challenging the dominant culture that creates that pain to begin with. Hence, what we defy is not only how we view the event but, more importantly, the dominant power structure, the patriarchy itself. When we defy the very process that tells us how to perceive, and challenge any forms of perceiving that support the status quo, it can no longer control us and cause us pain.

But before we begin to be fully committed to perceiving in defiant ways, we must always remember that perception, even when it is defiant, is still just a mirage.[34] I want to digress for a moment here to clarify the concept of perception as a mirage: that perception has no truth or essence, is always transient,[35] and can be "deceptive but [still] nonerroneous."[36] Perception as transient means that our perception can never be absolute because the thing we perceive is always changing; it is "episodic and relational" and does not have "stable physical properties."[37] When we see things or people as having a fixed essence, we will tend to cling to the idea that what we see, feel, or perceive is true. But because the object of our perception keeps changing—it is impermanent—and how we perceive it may shift depending on various factors, including our moods, whatever our perception of it is at a particular moment cannot be deemed as *the* truth.

Perception can be unreliable and deceptive, but it can still be nonerroneous. This means that although the appearance of a perception/mirage is deceptive, we cannot simply dismiss it as being false, because our sensory apparatus clearly registers its "presence."[38] Perhaps an example that has often been used by various philosophers may once again be useful here: someone who is color-blind has a limitation when it comes to perceiving certain colors outside their particular range of vision. This does not mean that what the person sees is wrong. Rather, it merely suggests that one's sensory apparatus of perception is limited and that what is being perceived may fall outside "the range of the sensory apprehension."[39] Similarly, our perception is shaped by our limited sensory apparatus, which has been disciplined in a certain way. There is a "range" of perceptive possibilities that limits our access to fully grasping what happens.[40] In this sense, perception may be deceptive and therefore unreliable, but its unreliability is not caused by its erroneous state.

To return to our conversation about an alternative process to perceiving, I would argue that the first step to challenging docile perception is to stop it in its track. When a perception emerges, and that perception is docile (i.e., a perception that we are accustomed to producing because that is how we are taught to perceive, and a perception that reflects the dominant thoughts of our culture), we need to practice "the art of non-reaction."[41] As the abbot and chief meditation master of Meetirigala Nissarana Vanaya Forest Monastery in Sri Lanka, Venerable Uda Eriyagama Dhammajīva Mahā Thero, elaborates, "Observe life's processes fully, from the beginning, the middle and to the end. When the whole episode is witnessed, a decision is unnecessary. It is when we just see the middle that we react and rush to a decision. . . . There is no rush to arrive at a decision. Instead, one remains in the present moment, unmoved by the projections created by perception."[42] Thus, rather than perceiving in the way that culture, social milieu, and history teach us to perceive, we simply observe and stay aware of the mirage and trickery that is taking place during the process of perception.[43] To be able to catch our docile perception as it happens and to not react to it is the first step to defying it.

Once we stop it in its tracks, we can then resist docile perception by questioning it. The next time we feel sad, hurt, or pained because of our perception, we can pause and ponder: Why did I perceive it in that way? Where did I learn to perceive it that way? What limits my perception or my range of perceptive possibilities? How does my perception create the pain I am feeling? Who benefits from my way of perceiving it this way? Whose interests does it serve? How does my perception function to uphold the dominant ideology? How can I perceive differently and/or defiantly? Whose perception is this? Here, I am not suggesting that we identify a person—this is not about "mine," "yours," or "theirs" or a particular subject's perception but rather, it is about recognizing that this perception is a function of a subjectivity that is historically and discursively disciplined to perceive in a certain way. This then allows us to evoke the Buddhist's sense of "nonself" or "nonbeing" and understand that there is no "authentic" subject/perceiver behind this perception to begin with. All subjectivities are a function of discourse and ideology.

This line of thinking follows in the footsteps of historian Joan Scott. I agree with Scott that "it is not individuals who have experience, but subjects who are constituted through experience."[44] However, she and I have different emphases in that for Scott, experience is considered as "a linguistic event," and "the question then becomes how to analyze language."[45] In this chapter, my purpose in raising the issue about perception is not registered only at the level of language but also at the somatic and sensory level of the *process* and *pattern of perception*. That there is a pattern in how we perceive that reflects the dominant and larger historical and cultural contexts within which a particular perception can emerge is what I call "docile perception."

Let us return, one last time, to the moment when I figured out why Renzo persisted in staying at that specific retreat. To defy docile perception, I need to first pause and remind myself that whatever perception I have about Renzo is a mere mirage and therefore unreliable and questionable. Beginning from this understanding would allow me to take a step back and not be invested in insisting that my story/perception is truer than his—neither perception is *the truth*. Then, I need to be aware that I am perceiving from a subjectivity that exists within a dominant discourse. In this case, my subjectivity is that of a jealous woman/partner, within a dominant discourse of a monogamous heterosexual romantic relationship.

Next, I need to defy perceiving from the "jealous woman" subjectivity. A woman who is constantly jealous and untrusting of others is easy to control. This is how patriarchy pins us down with its merciless claws. Occupying my time and thoughts by obsessively thinking about what he does with other women or whom he sexually desires; sneaking around and scrolling through his phone to see whom he sends text messages to (rather than spending time on my own research project or my community); excessively taking workshops in pursuit of the ultimate sexual techniques that I can master to keep him happy (rather than exploring what brings me pleasure and understanding how sexism operates in the very intimate space of our bedroom); or constantly purchasing new sexy lingerie even as I have yet to wear the last set I bought (rather than using the money to invest in my own financial wellness or that of my family's and community's)—this is how patriarchy controls me.[46]

Because defiant perception is not just about changing my own way of perceiving but also about challenging the power structure,[47] I would therefore also need to engage Renzo and invite him to see himself critically as a subjectivity that is created within a patriarchal discourse and challenge it. (I admit that this is a harder task that I do not always know how to do.) Moreover, since conversations about romantic relationships often happen beyond the people involved, and may include family members, friends, and therapists, we must therefore resist the urge to project arrogant/loving/docile perception when sharing our stories or giving romance-related advice to others. Remember, when we share our story/ advice in a certain way, we are teaching others a script for how to feel, think, and behave toward the other/event. Thus, it is important that we use these spaces of conversations as sites where we can practice to perceive in defiant ways.

To move beyond docile perception is to pause, question, and defy the perception that we are feeling at that moment as the event unfolds and render it unreliable. It is *not* to then rush into another, more positive, happier perception. Rather, it is to understand how that very perception is a form of disciplined perception that may perpetuate existing power dynamics, and to resist being implicated in the maintenance of the status quo. *To refuse to feel hurt when others try to intentionally wound us to keep/make us docile is to defy the power structure and reclaim our power.*

The bottom line here is this: pain has a way of making us docile. It is the most effective and affective disciplinary tool. Bullies aim to control us by hurting us (physically and/or emotionally), thereby using pain as a disciplinary tool. Perceiving in ways that hurt us will perpetuate our docility. As an instrument of docility, pain works not only at the level of the wound itself but also at the level of the process of making sense of it (the perception). Once we question our docile perception, our way of experiencing and carrying pain will then inevitably shift. The logic here is that once we are no longer carrying the pain the way that we did, we will have a better chance at resisting docile perception and becoming more defiant in our perception.

Thus, this cycle of perception and pain needs to be broken: docile perception often contributes to pain, and pain causes us to perceive in docile ways. Once we learn and practice alternative modes of perceiving, we can be liberated from the hold of our own perception that is hurting us, and we can then carry pain in a different way, or, depending on the kind of pain we have been carrying, we may be able to drop the pain altogether.

Certainly, we cannot stop perceiving. It is our life and survival mechanism. However, we do not have to automatically believe that what we perceive is true or reliable. The mere fact that we perceive it as such does not mean it is the truth. We also do not need to question each and every one of our perceptions either. But when a perception leads us to feeling pain, perhaps we may want to take a moment to pause, question that perception, and defy it. We can recite the mantra: this perception is painful to me; how can I perceive differently, in ways that do not hurt me more, and instead, reclaim my power and challenge the dominant power?

I hope it is clear that my theoretical intention and intervention with this chapter is to propose and point out how cognitive and affective processes of perception involve disciplining, regulating, and supervising the very process of perceiving, which reflects and supports the dominant ideology—the docile perception.[48] It is these *disciplining* processes that make perception "docile" and hence unreliable, and may even create more pain. It follows, then, that if docile perception is often found at the center of our unwarranted pain, we need to unlearn docile perception and unchain ourselves from the usual way we have been taught to perceive.

What I hope the readers will truly grasp after reading this chapter is how perception is not a private thought or something that is personal. Rather, it is deeply influenced by the dominant ideology of the time, and serves its interests instead of our well-being. It therefore often leads to pain, unless we are part of the dominant group it aims to serve.

This chapter thus functions as an invitation for the readers to be self-reflective in thinking about how and why we perceive the way that we do and the consequences of such docile perception, and, more importantly, how we can cultivate a different, more defiant perception that challenges power and the status quo. Eventually, it is only by tearing down the oppressive power that we will truly be liberated, not only in our perception but also in how we carry and relate to pain, and live our lives.

4

How Can I Work with My Body to Process Pain?

When I feel depressed, I register it as my body being held prisoner by the heaving pain. It is as if the pain physically chained my body to my bed. But it also feels as though my pain is being held hostage by my body. Even when I desperately want to push the pain out of my body, the body knows how to block every viable escape route I can think of. My body and my pain, as it seems, like to bring each other down to the ground, until the rock bottom is hit hard and raw.

Then, something usually happens that can unchain the bind between my body and my pain. Over a decade ago, as I was going through one of the most painful heartbreaks of my life, a dear friend suggested that I jog. So jog I did. So excessively, in fact, that not only did I *feel* lighter but I literally *became* lighter, about twenty-five pounds lighter to be exact, within a period of one month. (I would not recommend losing weight at that unhealthy rate or getting your heart nastily broken. The latter is tricky, I know.) Luckily, though, the process of resetting the relationship between my body and my pain does not always involve excessive exercise. Oftentimes, it is simply about turning to cakes, chocolates, and caramels until the sadness feels soft and moist in my mouth.

What I did not realize until I was writing this book was that what eventually shattered the shackle that bound my body with my pain was my ability to re/turn to and work with the body. Thus, if in the previous chapter I paid attention to the mind/perception, in this chapter I shift the focus to the body. I want to tell a story about my experiences of staying at a meditation ashram in Nepal and practicing a new meditation method that guides me to work with my body and helps me feel and process my pain (rather than numb the pain, which was how I usually dealt with it). However, what makes this meditation technique unique is how it returns me to the body by way of working *without the story* (through the gibberish method). Hence, my conversation in this chapter, which focuses on the body, is couched within this framework of foregoing the story.

## No-Mind Therapy Meditation: Can You Cry without the Story?

Osho Tapoban ashram is located in Nagarjun Hills Forest Reserve, about nine kilometers from Kathmandu, Nepal. The center has scheduled daily meditations that run from 7:00 a.m. until 10:00 or 11:00 p.m. Meditators are free to choose whichever session they want to participate in. All meditation sessions, except special programs such as the no-mind therapy, are included in the price. The cost of my deluxe room/meals/ meditations was 35 USD/day. (As a context, in 2017, when I visited, the minimum monthly salary in Nepal was about 67 USD.)[1] The center has different fee schedules depending on which country the person comes from (for local participants, the fee can be as low as 7 USD/day). They also have a volunteer program where meditators can stay for free in exchange for their service/work. The no-mind therapy runs almost every month, from the first to the seventh. It costs an additional 70 USD for the week. I stayed at the ashram from August 30 to September 14, 2017. On most days, I spent seven hours meditating, including the two hours/day of no-mind therapy.

When I went to Nepal, I had been practicing meditation for twelve years. In 2005, I moved to Vancouver, Canada, where I lived within walking distance of community centers that offered meditation classes. After I began to take meditation classes, I became intrigued by different modalities of mindfulness and learned various meditation techniques, from visualization to zazen. In Canada, I also went to a variety of classes on emotional freedom techniques and shamanic drumming circles, and even got certifications (levels 1, 2, and 3) in Reiki healing. In 2014, I did a ten-day Vipassana silent meditation in Calgary, Canada, during which we were not allowed to speak or engage (even through eye contact) with other meditators. During the Vipassana retreat, I learned that intentional silence could become an empowering and healing space. All of these healing modalities had helped me improve my overall well-being and prepared me for the no-mind therapy in Nepal, which then propelled me to further shift my relationship with pain in significant ways.

No-mind therapy was created by Osho (born Chandra Mohan Jain in India, 1931–1990). He was a philosophy professor at Raipur Sanskrit College and the University of Jabalpur. He later resigned and became one of the most influential and controversial spiritual leaders and thinkers of his time. He was considered radical for his teachings, which challenged established religions and governments and even questioned the existence of God. He moved to the United States in 1981 and with his followers built a commune in Oregon. Following a series of scandals, he was detained and deported by the American government a few years later. Many other countries refused to grant him entry. He then returned to India and further expanded what is now called the Osho International Meditation Retreat in Pune, India. Other meditation/retreat centers that followed his teachings were organized locally across different regions and countries, including the one in Nagarjun, Nepal, that I visited.

No-mind therapy was one of Osho's signature active meditations. It is a two-hour sequenced meditation. The first hour is dedicated to releasing all emotions repressed in the body. For this step, meditators are encouraged to practice gibberish, to make noises with no words, such as "a-u-o-a-a-o-i-u-o-a," so that buried emotions can resurface. Gibberish becomes a pathway to induce our emotions. The second step for no-mind therapy is lying down in a corpse pose for thirty minutes, in silence. The third step is to sit and meditate for thirty minutes. The premise for this sequenced meditation is that it is only after releasing the body's emotions through active bodily movements and gibberish practices during the first hour that meditation with silent mind is possible.[2] Gibberish is deemed important because it is a tool to get meditators to the deepest, most buried emotion that is registered outside the con-

scious mind. I consider this gibberish (nonstory) significant for processing our pain because through this practice of accessing emotion beyond
language, we can bypass the patriarchal discourses and emotional hegemony through which we make sense of the world and are made to feel a
certain way, and instead weaken their hold in our lives.

When the meditation teacher introduced us to this gibberish/
releasing-of-emotions technique, he likened this method to what in
Western psychology is called "catharsis." "Catharsis" comes from the
Greek word "*katharsis*," meaning "purging or cleansing, a release or
evacuation of something."[3] The core principle of catharsis is that repressed negative emotions may become psychologically harmful, and
therefore we need to purge these emotions by way of acting them out
and bearing witness to them.[4]

Catharsis can also be understood as a release that is experienced
through others. In narratives or plays/theater performances, catharsis
is often expressed as "a power of vicariousness, of being elsewhere (in
another time or place), of imagining differently, experiencing the world
through the eyes of strangers."[5] That is, when pain is too unbearable for
a person to experience it directly, it can be relived from a safe distance
through other people's experiences.[6] Writers and poets are important
in this way because their writings help induce the readers' process of
catharsis through their stories.

Early theorists such as John Dollard, Leonard Doob, Neal Miller, O.
H. Mowrer, and Robert Sears view catharsis as productive because it can
decrease the possibility of future aggression. Later studies, however, have
challenged this, and instead show that exercising catharsis can lead to
increased aggression.[7] These differences may, according to psychologists
Konrad Bresin and Kathryn Gordon, be related to how scholars may
conflate aggression with violence. According to them, there is a difference between aggression, defined as "behaviors that increase the relative
social dominance of an individual," and violence, "the use of dominance
to cause severe psychological or physical harm to others."[8] It is aggression that catharsis encourages, not violence.

There is also a difference between "Western" catharsis and Osho's catharsis. Osho's catharsis uses gibberish to resurface buried emotions so that they can be released. That is, rather than going to their pain via stories, meditators are encouraged to go to their pain via nonstories. Thus, during the first step of the no-mind therapy meditation, gibberish is used as a way to bypass the mind and invoke the affective body to call forth the emotions that are buried deep within the subconscious mind. When emotions surface, meditators are encouraged to let their bodies do what they need to do: cry, wail, scream, punch the pillow, or make whatever gestures the body wants to make. The body becomes "an expressive, corporeal language."[9] In evoking the body, this meditation technique uses the body as "an active agent in remembering history."[10] The body is considered as an archive, "a museum, the site of collection of memories. Through the body, one can recall the past and remember the traumatic pain."[11] Gibberish is thus touted in this ashram as a method that allows the body to recall such a traumatic, painful past, *without the story.*

The only, and important, rule of this technique at the first stage is this: when the mind starts to create stories about the emotions, the meditators need to drop those stories. Meditators need to go back to the body, the emotions, and the gibberish practice. By letting out all of the suppressed emotions, meditators will empty their mind and body fully. Then, they are ready for the second and third steps of meditating. No-mind therapy becomes a way to embody and express these emotions in a safe environment.

To clarify, I am not arguing that story does not matter. Stories *do* matter. They can function as tools to explore and examine what it means to be human.[12] They can be helpful in providing us with a way to make sense of our lives and emotions, and for other people to understand us.[13] They even have the power to heal.[14]

What I am arguing is that stories at times may fail to take us into the realm of pain that is registered *affectively* in the body, let alone to free us from it. Feminist discourse, for instance, may be useful in helping us understand pain, the structural and patriarchal conditions that contribute to that pain, but not in pushing us to experience, express, and transcend pain fully. At times, feminism can become a narrow way of seeing, feeling, and understanding our pain, or even the world. Thus, I propose that we return to the body and consider nonstory—gibberish spaces—to help us process our pain.

I want to digress for a moment here to highlight that it is not a coincidence that it was in Nepal that I began to think about the importance of gibberish. Being in a country where I could not speak the language, I was aware of how not having access to what other meditators were talking about during breakfast/lunch/dinner/evening celebrations/breaks, etc., allowed me to be increasingly aware of the potential usefulness of nonstory in our lives. In other words, and to return to my research method, my transnational travel and autoethnography matter in helping me to understand the connection between the limitation of language and the processing of pain, and to arrive at this knowledge.[15]

In this book, I frame gibberish as an embodied mode of expressing emotions without the stories. Here, I do not mean embodiment to be "precultural."[16] Rather, I offer gibberish as an aural, affective, and somatic mode of communication: a way of speaking that is not understood by the self or others. Gibberish can therefore be apprehended as chaos in narrative, and as such it creates a rupture in legible discursive spaces. Although there are different forms of gibberish expressions, such as sound poetry or other nonsense verse, the only gibberish practice that I discuss here is the no-mind therapy meditation technique practiced at the specific ashram that I visited.

## My Experiences: What Gibberish as a Meditation Technique Does to My Pain

It was fifteen minutes before eleven o'clock in the morning and I showed up in the same maroon robe/dress that all meditators had to wear. I also had a maroon blindfold in my pocket that we had to use during these active meditations. I was nervous and skeptical. But Swami Krishna, the meditation teacher, had a calm demeanor that made me feel relaxed right away. He began the session by asking us to come forward to hear his explanation about the meditation, if we never had done this type before. I, along with other new students, approached him. It was my first day of no-mind therapy, although it was my second day doing meditation at the ashram. I had been attending a few other meditation sessions there and slowly learned and adopted new meditation techniques.

Although there were about forty people that week (not counting the people who work and volunteer at the ashram, who also joined some of the sessions) who participated in other meditation sessions throughout the day, only seven people, including myself, were doing the no-mind therapy. There were two participants from China, and four from Nepal, two male and five female participants. Perhaps having to pay an additional 70 USD for the week of no-mind therapy was a deterrent. Some visitors came for three or four days only, making it harder to join a week-long session. However, it is worthy of note that because the retreat center had a sliding-scale fee structure and volunteer opportunities to stay at the center, there were more locals joining the program overall, compared to the other retreats I participated in.

Swami explained the sequence of the meditation, first in English, then in Nepali. After he was done, we went back to our mattresses. Each of us had a set consisting of a thin mattress, a white bed sheet, and a pillow to punch to express anger. "Ready? Let's stand up and get started," Swami said with a smile. He had the kind of smile that soothed me. He pulled back his long, dark hair, and pressed the play button on his smartphone to start the music.

It was not exactly music as such. Nor was it calm or meditative. It was loud music with fast-paced drumming and chaotic screaming in the background. The hectic voices of men and women screaming, laughing, and crying, which were used to evoke participants' screams, resembled the way the laugh track in TV sitcoms is used to induce viewers' laughter. I began to feel as if this whole therapy was a scam, a cult practice of some sort. I doubted my decision to be there. I wanted to leave. Within seconds, however, I could not even hear the music. All I heard was other participants shouting, crying, and hitting their pillows violently. Shocked, afraid, and confused, I resorted to what Swami had told us: "If you can't scream, don't just stay silent. When you stay silent you will absorb other people's negative emotions. Just do gibberish." I started practicing gibberish.

"Aiueuioiuuueieoeieueieoeieuoieueoiueoiueoieuoeiuouaaiusoauoui-uaoaiuoiauoiauoe," I began with a soft and tentative voice, moving my jaw chaotically in all directions.

Other participants were shouting even louder at the top of their lungs. I heard someone wailing with so much pain that I could feel her pain as my own. As the room was flooded with bold and boisterous emotions, I began to do gibberish in a louder voice. I allowed myself to be consumed with the strangeness happening around and within me and let my body do what it needed to do. As I was doing gibberish, my eyes started to feel warm, my chest felt heavy, and my throat became raw. I felt deep stabbing sadness at the center of my heart as it began to move upward toward my throat, then to my mouth. As it reached my mouth, I started to sob. And then I wailed. For no particular reason. At no one in particular.

Random images started to pop into my head. The deception, betrayal, and abandonment that had become a pattern in my love life began to appear one after the other, as in a parade. As the saying goes, different faces, different places, but the story remained the same: devastating heartbreak, mostly mine. Then, images of my father and his string of mistresses appeared. My father had been an absent father in my life. His absence left a huge, gaping hole in my heart in the shape of a longing that I dared not trace. I felt a chronic sense of unworthiness, of being unloved, and of being unseen. I felt completely alone, lonely, and abandoned. Hopeless. I curled up my body as I cried louder. I wanted to soothe my own pain. The intensity of pain emptied me of all my tears.

At that moment, I remembered what Swami had said earlier: "Don't think." When we think, he said, we get stuck in that pain. We cannot

go deeper into the pain. We cannot resurface and release all the emotions that need to be expressed. So, I went back to doing gibberish,
bypassing the mind, letting go of the story. As I stayed with my body,
with my emotions, I began to howl like a wolf. It is as if I had just gotten shot and was waiting for the moment of death to arrive. Each time
a story would pop up, as soon as I realized it was happening, I would
go back to practicing gibberish to drop the story. To help me let go of
the story, I used a visual trick of imagining the story or whatever image
appeared in my mind falling onto the ground and evaporating at the
same time.

Then, minutes later, I suddenly felt enraged, and my howling turned
into a wild beast's roar. Pain and rage colonized my body. I was yell-
ing, screaming, and shrieking. Suddenly, my body made some stabbing
gestures. My anger was directed toward patriarchy and the patriarch in
my family. And as stories about how badly the patriarch had treated
me came back, I shook my head to clear those stories one more time
and went back to feeling the rise and fall of all of the body's emotions.
And the cycle continued: each time a different image popped up, and
stories about the situation followed, I dropped them as soon as I caught
myself doing the storifying. In this sense, gibberish can be understood
as a self-reflective mode of being in the body that provokes buried stories to resurface. Nonetheless, it is our faithfulness to the nonstory, our
persistence in crying without the story, so to speak, our really being in
our body and not our mind, that can take us further and further into the
process of transcending pain. In other words, for as long as we entertain
the stories, we will be trapped in the pain.

One hour of screaming, mining the well of repressed emotions and
expressing them with such force and intensity, sounds like a long time.
But when the bell rang, I felt that even an hour was not enough to express all of the emotions that were buried deep within me. I felt my
body was just getting warmed up and that I still wanted to roar, wail,
and punch. Yet, the moment had come when we had to completely stop
and lie down in the savasana position (corpse pose) for thirty minutes.

As I lay there on a thin mattress, my tears began to dry up, and my breathing became slower. I gradually felt calmer. I was exhausted, yet I felt very peaceful. Slowly and gently, I was drifting away to that sweet spot of tranquility, that perfect moment right before I fall asleep, and I floated there for a while, enjoying the feeling of serenity, of just being, of nothingness. And before I knew it, Swami rang the bell, alerting us that it was now time for sitting meditation. By that time, after going through this sequence of activities, I became silent with my thoughts. I meditated with vast openness in my heart, mind, body, and soul. I felt relaxed, as if the pain had been transcended, as if I had given the pain some wings with which to fly. I felt liberated. Perhaps it was the knowledge that I can go deep into my own pain, and yet still stand strong and not die, that set me free. That was perhaps the moment when I could truly extend my hand to embrace pain, to shift my relationship with it.

Every day for seven days, we started the same way, with an hour-long gibberish session to release all repressed emotions, and then savasana and sitting meditation for the second hour. During the seven days of the program, my experience varied. I was releasing not only anger, sadness, and pain but also joy and laughter.

On the third day, for example, when the music was on and Swami instructed us to begin, I started doing the usual gibberish to induce whatever feelings my body wanted to express that day. And that morning, I wanted to yell. So, I yelled, screamed, and roared. Loudly. By then, I felt more comfortable shouting.

Images of my father and his mistresses started to come back once more. This time the image was of another recent event when my father's longtime mistress demanded that he sell our family house and small boutique hotel so she could have access to the money before my aging and sick father died. He complied, forcing my mother to sign the papers. I screamed as loud as I could, trying to reach for the lever of release that I had yet to find. My anger was boiling beyond its hottest temperature. Stories began to flow into the volcanic mountains of my mindscape. Then, an image appeared of my father telling my mother that after he sold the properties he would take *all* of the money. The realization that my father was a bully, an emotionally abusive man, made me question: If I am my father's daughter, then, what does that make me? But then, I caught myself getting stuck in my own anger and shame. Even though there were more questions I wanted to ask and justice I wanted to seek, I let go of these stories and let my emotions take the driver's seat. And I went along for the bumpy ride.

Suddenly, out of the blue, I felt the strong urge to laugh out loud, as if there were a ridiculous hilarity bug that had bitten me. I had no clue what was funny—there was no story—but something seemed so comical that my laughter became uncontrollable. I wondered if that meant that there was some repressed laughter or joy in me. I laughed until my stomach was in pain, tears coming down my cheeks, once again.

Then, to my surprise, I started humming the soundtrack to *Twilight Zone*—one of my favorite television shows when I was a child. I then began to sit on my knees and found myself rocking back and forth. I curled up into a ball, hugging myself. I started humming and singing a lullaby in a high-pitched voice like those ghosts in scary movies. I had goose bumps and started to feel afraid, not quite sure of what, perhaps of myself because at that point I felt as if I had lost control. I was worried that I had become completely crazy and was not going to be able to control my emotions anymore. But that thought, too, I quickly brushed away, clearing the space for nonstory.

Then, different images came up in my mind: first, of two white persons. One was a little girl and the other was her mother. The mother was telling her dying little girl, "I love you, my love. Go to sleep, my love." I was not sure who they were although later that evening, I remembered that I had been grieving over the loss of my friend's two-year-old daughter. Then, an image of my late grandmother came up. She was my go-to person, my compass, my strong feminist role model. She was my biggest supporter. When she passed away, a few months after 9/11 and immigration rules for citizens of Muslim countries (including Indonesia, where I came from) tightened, I was in the United States. Not wanting to risk not being able to return, I missed her funeral. I regretted that decision and the missed opportunity of saying goodbye one last time and thanking her for what she had done for me. In my mind, I saw her being buried, her face so peaceful. I could feel my entire body trembling. I was sobbing uncontrollably. As I started singing "Amazing Grace," the feelings of sadness became even more overwhelming. At that moment, I could feel a big boulder pressing on my chest and a tornado sucking the consciousness out of me, making me feel light, dizzy, and as though I was going to faint. I could feel explosives going off at the very core of my heart. My heart was beyond broken. My pain was simply unbearable. I was experiencing a level of sorrow and sadness, of loss, loneliness, and lunacy that I had never accessed before. And at that moment, my sobbing, bawling, and wailing seemed minuscule in comparison to whatever feelings were moving me and moving in/outside of me. Even as I write this chapter and try to access those emotions in order to find words to describe the intense feelings, I fail.

Moments later, the sound of the singing bowl was vibrating throughout the room, alerting us that one hour was over. I slowly transitioned to the savasana pose, and then eventually to sitting meditation.

Although my experiences would vary each day, collectively they allowed me to process, access, and transcend my emotions. These experiences helped me understand the limitation of words, stories, and feminist theories in engaging with pain differently. That is, when I allow my body to express what it wants, when I can feel the feelings without the story, something inside me propels me to move in a direction that I had never gone in before. As sociologist Michal Pagis argues in her analysis of Vipassana, a different form of meditation that practices complete silence, "In meditation, in order to know oneself, one does not speak either with another or with oneself. Instead, self-knowledge is anchored in bodily sensations."[17] Similarly, meditation technique, such as the no-mind therapy that relies on the body and foregoes the stories, is crucial because when I let only narratives and stories guide me to where and what I want to feel, I am not able to tap into those other, deeper feelings. I become trapped in those stories.

Stories may only take us to the portal of our emotional archive. But nonstory may take us further to the affective realm of emotions that the mind has forgotten, that memory has abandoned, and that consciousness has suppressed. Nonstory bypasses the discourse, the cognition.

After my one-week experience of no-mind therapy, I was able to replay those moments of pain in my life without feeling their sting. There were no feelings attached to what happened. That is, the way I felt toward my father had shifted. There was no anger toward him. Again, this does not mean that I have forgotten and condoned what happened or will stop working toward the end of patriarchy, which contributes to the culture that encourages men like my father to behave in ways that are hurtful toward the women in his life. However, my relationship to pain shifted in significant ways. I truly felt peaceful. I would liken my blissful feeling to those first moments of falling in love, when my eyes shine brighter and my heart cheers loudly, but without the obsessive feeling toward the object of love, because in this case, there was no one in particular I had fallen in love with.[18]

I want to emphasize here that it is our capacity to cry, so to speak, *without* the story, that is key in processing pain with our body. When we can cry without the story, when we can truly feel and honor the presence of pain and transcend it—not because we will our mind to it but because that is where the body takes us—that is when pain/emotions can liberate us. We are free. This freedom comes from letting go of the patriarchal language, discourses, and systems of meaning that have been the true prison in our lives.

Thus, if for feminist philosopher Elaine Scarry, pain causes "an immediate reversion to a state anterior to language, to the sounds and cries a human being makes before language is learned,"[19] for me, the no-mind therapy allows me to intentionally and purposefully let go of language and embrace the nonstory so that I can dig deeper into pain and transcend how I carry it. I learn to hear (with) the body without it having to speak to me through "a language of symptoms."[20] In other words, unlike Scarry, I consider gibberish not as a mere effect of pain but rather as a tool to process pain more deeply.

## Gibberish and the Need to Work with the Body and without the Story

To return to the book's reframing of pain as an anamorphic apparatus, I want to assert here that had I not used pain as a tool with which to see differently, I would have not understood the importance of working simultaneously with the body and without the story to process pain in our lives. The pain that I was carrying with me as I was traveling and practicing the no-mind therapy allows me to theorize differently about what it means to take seriously the phenomenon of pain embodiment (e.g., how pain can at times be repressed or lodged deeply in the body affectively, but not necessarily cognitively) and to be faithful to nonstory in order to transcend pain.

In embracing the nonstory, specifically the gibberish practice during the no-mind therapy, I want to highlight how existing modes of processing pain that use written or spoken words in ways that others or the self can understand have limited us in going deeper into our pain.[21] In this sense, language functions as a barrier to reaching and resurfacing long-buried emotions, especially those emotions that are registered precognitively. This is the case because language and specific discourses (feminist discourses included) can operate as maps and routes that orient and direct us toward certain familiar emotional spaces, but not others.

When we let go of language—that is, practice gibberish—we can feel and explore our emotions without the map (discourses/stories) and venture into intriguing and uncharted emotional spaces that we would have otherwise not visited. In other words, gibberish frees us from these maps, and hence from predictable and predetermined emotional destinations, and from formulas for how to transcend them. In this way, gibberish provides us with a distinct mode of engagement with pain as it takes us deeper into our pain via nonstory.

Let's take my experience to clarify this point. During the meditation, when I saw an image, a memory, or an experience in my mind's eye, and recited stories that were attached to these experiences, these stories became a map charting how and where my feelings would go. These stories convince me of what and how to feel, and whom to blame. If I did not drop these stories, I would be stuck in them, in that pain, and in my own anger. (Think here of the dominant script discussed in chapter 3.) I would not be able to go deeper into other feelings this anger was sitting on top of, nor grasp what these layers of feelings meant for *me*— what underlying fear or emotions *within me* made me feel the way that I did. I might not be able to see how my feelings toward my mother, for instance, had also caused me pain, or how my mother's relationship with my father had shaped the contour of my own romantic relationships. Even this, the narrative of how my mother's/father's romantic relationship influences my own, *is a story*. I have been so good at believing in this story and others like it that they limit how I experience my emotions and my life in general. To transform my relationship with pain, my body, and myself, I need to drop this story. I need to expose, explore, and express my pain without the story.

Moreover, if I felt the anger toward my father to the point that I wanted to hurt him (expressed by the stabbing gestures during my no-mind therapy session), and such a feeling made me feel bad because I knew I was not supposed to feel that way, and then I censored my feelings, I would not have been able to access deeper buried emotions and feel all emotions to the fullest. I would be trapped at this level of emotion.

Gibberish practice thus helps us reach those sensations lodged in the body that are registered affectively, that our cognitive mind cannot quite comprehend even when we feel them in the present moment. It helps us get at what is troubling us at a deeper level. Thus, we need to forego stories, discourses, and language in processing pain, especially when they function as prohibitive borders that stop us from going further with our emotions.

To consider gibberish as a way to reach repressed emotions in the body by bypassing language is to shed light on the long-standing problem of language as "a reliable system."[22] Author George Orwell points out, "Linguistic construction is an ideological process that carries with it a legacy of centuries of cultural and political violence."[23] Immigrants often find that language "betrays" them "on a continual basis."[24] If language is always implicated within violent ideological processes, then shouldn't we, as feminists, find ways to speak beyond language, to bypass language, to create spaces outside ideologies and discourses that could better help us engage with emotions and pain?

Indeed, in their efforts to bring down patriarchy, poststructuralist feminists have challenged the use of male-dominated language. Some scholars, such as Hélène Cixous and Monique Wittig, uphold the idea that because language itself is already and always patriarchal, to reject such a masculine language therefore is to resist.[25] Following this trajectory, gibberish that is used to induce and resurface buried emotions that are then expressed also in gibberish form (with no story attached, even as it tries to sneak into our mind) can therefore be considered a powerful feminist tool as it bypasses the patriarchal language within which we make sense of our emotions and learn how/what to feel.

Simply put, the gibberish technique is crucial in processing pain because it allows us to evade patriarchal language in doing so. It is an appeal to process pain differently while not putting patriarchy once again at the center of our stories nor using patriarchal language to express our pain. I would even propose that it be one of the answers to literary scholar Ananya Kabir's call that we find other ways to express trauma that can "bypass the pitfalls of the chain of connections between language, narrative and realistic representation."[26] Simultaneously, to practice gibberish and return to the body and the body's mode of accessing repressed emotions beyond patriarchal language is to heed transnational feminist theorist M. Jacqui Alexander's advice that "if healing work is a call to remember and remembering is embodied, then we would want to situate the body centrally in this healing complex."[27] Indeed, working with the body and foregoing the story are among the central feminist practices that this book proposes we do to process and carry pain differently in our lives.

Practicing gibberish can also be considered a feminist practice as it takes up a space, an actual physical space, for a person must claim a space to do gibberish, and to speak up—although without a story—and to occupy a sonic space nonetheless. In other words, we make our voices heard in space but not in ways that can be understood by others. It is a space where the body is given permission and even encouraged to feel and express whatever it needs to, until it is emptied of its repressed emotions. (One of the problems I have in practicing no-mind therapy/ gibberish in my daily life is not being able to find a space where I can scream and wail as madly and loudly as I need to, without having the neighbors call a cop on me.) In this way, gibberish space can function as a third space. It moves us beyond the binary spaces of silence, which has its value,[28] and voice, where the ability to speak up and be legible for others is emphasized.[29]

In defying the binary, gibberish space can be considered subversive. In gibberish, the point of articulation is not to communicate with others (to make the self understood), to make sense of one's own life, or to connect with others. The emphasis on the need to understand or on understanding itself is what the practice of gibberish challenges. By practicing gibberish, we insist that the point should not solely and always be about understanding, but rather, to access that which has been hidden even from ourselves because patriarchal ways of living, speaking, and thinking teach us to speak and express our emotions in a particular way that is not conducive to our well-being.

It may even be "healing" to create spaces of illegibility where we do not have to understand each other. Particularly in this digital and social media age, where the self is often constructed for the audience's/other's gaze, to practice gibberish—that is, to speak up but not with an audience in mind nor to be understood, and instead with the goal of excavating deeply buried emotions in order to release and transcend them—can indeed be both healing and subversive—it has the potential to challenge the status quo.

In closing, I want to reiterate that the point of this chapter is to provide one example of how *I* worked with the body and without the story to process my pain. I do not, in any way, argue that this is *the* only way to process pain. There is room for silences and voices, as well as gibberish/nonstory sonic spaces. By detailing the practice of no-mind therapy, I want to show how gibberish becomes a space that allows *me* to carry pain differently. It leads me to profoundly transcend both the feelings and the understandings of pain. It also allows me to grasp how gibberish can become a safe and potentially subversive space where nonstory matters and where deeper feelings can resurface in order to be experienced, expressed, and eventually transcended. It is my hope that after reading this chapter, the readers will feel more compelled to process pain in their lives by working with the body and without the story, in whichever form of embodied practice may fit them best.

5

# How Can I Practice Feminist Enchantment in My Everyday Life?

You'll need magic to make it out of here
—Ocean Vuong

And could you keep your heart in wonder at the daily miracles of your life, your pain would not seem less wondrous than your joy
—Kahlil Gibran

The two epigraphs that begin this chapter offer us a soothing, yet stirring poetic insight into the life of and with pain: they tell us we must weave magic and miracle into the fabric of our daily lives to survive. Indeed, I craft this chapter as being born/e out of and carrying this wisdom throughout its pages. I want to show how the magic of enchantment—more specifically, what I call "feminist enchantment"—can be an antidote to pain. By "antidote," I do not mean I have found a cure for the pain. Rather, I mean that I carry pain in ways that allow me to play and be playful with pain (even though it still exists), to dip in and out of pain, and to feel alive in the midst of it all. (Prior to practicing feminist enchantment and/or other techniques mentioned in this book, for instance, I often had to numb myself so I did not have to feel the pain, which is the opposite of feeling alive.)

I define "feminist enchantment" as an embodied feminist practice that connects us to ourselves, and connects our mind, body, and spirit to our surroundings—the materiality of the city or the place where we are at the moment.[1] (Remember, if the first question of the book focuses on the mind/perception, and the second question, on the body, the third question aims to connect the mind to the body and to its surround-ings/environment.) This enchantment practice is feminist in that it is rooted in feminist thought and embodiment,[2] and helps us reclaim our body, power, and agency. By doing so, we will then be able to carry pain differently.

Feminist enchantment involves three core practices: (1) forgetting, (2) embodying the erotic as a life force, and (3) bodily remembering of the body's natural state of being playful. To clarify these points, in the first part of the chapter, I will share my stories of traveling to places where I experienced feminist enchantment and my pain greatly dissipated (e.g., Ecuador, Iceland, and Spain). Then, in the second part of the chapter, I will turn to how enchantment can be found not only in spontaneous and scattered moments of awe (as will be discussed in the first part of the chapter) but also in moments of repetition with a twist. I will focus spe-cifically on the example of walking every day (the repetition) in Kotor and Madrid, but with each day exploring different routes or encounter-ing different enjoyment (with a twist), and how my pain waned as I was practicing feminist enchantment in these cities.

As a note of clarification: although travel may induce new bodily practices and enchantment, I do not argue that enchantment as an anti-dote to pain can only be practiced during travel. It is indeed travel that brings me to enchantment (and to the theories in this chapter and in this book) and that provides me with a shortcut, so to speak, to escape the pain in the here and now by traveling to a different place where such pain is "forgotten." But feminist enchantment is a daily practice that can be (and I encourage it to be) adopted anywhere, including at home.

To provide us with a context of pain that is chronically carried by my body, I must first disclose the nature of my autoimmune disease and chronic low back pain, whose intensity changes depending on where I travel and the state of my being enchanted.

## Body That Betrays: Autoimmune Disease and Chronic Low Back Pain

Our body is but a ticking time bomb. Pain is what makes the ticking palpable.

I was diagnosed with an autoimmune disease called Graves' disease (hyperthyroidism) when I was seventeen. When I was nineteen, I exhibited one of the symptoms of the disease: a goiter that made my neck look swollen, turning me into an easy target for teasing. It was embarrassing enough, or rather, I was embarrassed about my body enough, that I was desperate for surgery. Yet, at the time, my doctor did not think it would be safe for me to have surgery to remove it. I thence continued taking the medicine as prescribed. I also drank traditional herbs that my father told me would help me heal.

My father was a traditional healer—at least, some people would consider him as such. I did not really believe he had "gifts," although I had seen him perform the ritual in which he was possessed by the "spirit" who used his body as a medium to counsel and heal the person/patient who came to him for help. To treat my illness, my father had to meditate and fast until he received the answer to what could cure me, and then climb a mountain to a sacred spot to get the roots and herbs needed. I do not remember what the healing concoction was made of—I just remember its awful, bitter, nauseating taste. Yet, even after all of these efforts, my blood tests, TSH, T3, and T4, were still abnormal. I was put on methimazole indefinitely. The goiter, however, eventually shrank.

When I moved to the United States, my doctor recommended radioactive iodine therapy. It was a common treatment for my condition, with a possible side effect of experiencing hypothyroidism (which means that I would then have to take Synthroid for the rest of my life). I declined the treatment. I suppose I was stubborn. Or perhaps, I refused the treatment because I grew up in a culture and household where traditional herbs were considered medicine, and we were more suspicious than trusting of Western medicine.

After over fifteen years of taking my thyroid medication, I grew tired of taking the pills every day, and became worried about long-term side effects. I decided to wean myself off the medication, but continued to get a blood test every six months, per doctor's orders. When the blood tests and the doctor deemed it necessary that I go back to medication, I would. But then, after I felt better, I would take myself off the medication again, and the cycle continued. Because the results of my blood tests have mostly improved, I have been getting tested only once a year for almost a decade now. In the event that I started to feel fatigue for no reason, feel out of breath just walking across the street, experience faster heartbeat, or have extreme irritability/mood issues, I would then request to have the blood tests done earlier than scheduled. I have accepted the fact that I may have to do this for the rest of my life.

As if Graves' disease is not enough, I had to add to my list of chronic illness low back pain. The peak of my pain was summer 2007, just after I graduated from my doctoral program, when I was living in Vancouver, Canada. I was preparing to move to Atlanta to take a postdoctoral position. Surely, packing for a move could add to the back pain that I already had. However, about a week before my move, I took a level four solo kayaking workshop. A whole day of practicing solo rescue and carrying the kayak myself (and making the mistake of lifting with my back, instead of my knees) took a toll on my back. The following days, I could not even get up without assistance. Yet, somehow, I managed to fly to Atlanta. But I never really fully healed. Most mornings my back would be so stiff and sore that I had to slide sideways out of bed.

As my case and those of many others suggest, back pain is, in a sense, uncanny. It is "psychosomatic" in that to address it, we must pay attention to both the psychological and the "pathological somatic aspects" of the disease simultaneously.[3] Though it is often "mechanical in origin" and worsened by aging and injury, back pain requires psychological as well as mechanical approaches to address it.[4] In my case, I tried psychotherapy, acupuncture, physiotherapy, and chiropractic adjustments. I also practiced yoga and Pilates, and held my legs up the wall, which was supposed to help with my back pain. After years of practicing these measures to no avail, in 2013, I got an MRI, which showed mild degenerative disc disease and mild osteoarthritis of the facet joints of L5–S1. My physiotherapist was puzzled, as his treatment would have alleviated the pain caused by these issues. He then recommended that I see his colleague, who suggested an interventional radiology procedure. I refused that, but did purchase an expensive (but useless) undergarment that he said could ease my back pain. I also tried reversal table therapy and swimming, per his suggestions. I gave up tennis and all kinds of yoga (especially where I had to do forward folds and twists) except for yin yoga, as they would worsen my back pain. None of these efforts, however, seemed to completely heal me. My back pain, it seems, is as stubborn as I am.

Both my autoimmune disease and my low back pain are considered chronic pain. Geriatric nurse specialist Gudrun Gudmannsdottir and professor of nursing Sigridur Halldorsdottir define chronic pain ("the pain of khronos, time") as "persistent pain that has lasted for at least three months" and continues to exist even after it has "lost its warning functions and attends with psychosocial changes."[5] Chronic pain can come at any time, intermittently or persistently, and may be found in a specific location of the body/mind or felt radiating to different parts of the body.[6] Because chronic pain comes without warning and is uncontrollable, it can be perceived as "an intrusion of the outside into the body or as a betrayal of internal bodily stasis."[7] Indeed, my chronic pain often makes me feel betrayed by my own body.

What differentiates nonchronic from chronic pain is that in the case of chronic pain, the brain can produce the experience of pain.[8] For chronic pain, there is a "decreased sensory processing and enhanced emotional/cognitive processing of pain."[9] This means that in terms of chronic pain, negative emotions can make the sufferer feel more pain. The fact that chronic pain is "highly contextual" provides us with an opportunity to cultivate a more inspiring context in order to carry it in a more life-sustaining way.[10] Some of these techniques that have worked to alleviate chronic pain include "relaxation and imagery techniques" and "a cognitive-behavioral treatment."[11] To this list of effective methods that can help us shift how we carry (chronic) pain in our lives, I want to add the embodied daily practice of "feminist enchantment."

## Three Core Practices of Feminist Enchantment

*I traveled because I wanted to be in awe. I wanted to be wowed. I wanted to be bathed in the magnificent grandeur of the world, of something I cannot experience at home. I wanted to experience magic.* Feeling lost in the chaotic mess and loneliness of travel, I questioned why I needed to travel. And this was my answer.

When I read this answer during the process of writing this book, I caught a glimpse of my own naiveté. How could I, a grown woman, a researcher, talk about magic as if it were real? Is there such a thing as magic outside of movies and fairy tales? As I lingered and poked around the answer to why I travel, I began to see the need to deconstruct my answer, to trace its truth and transcend its meanings. It was this desire that led me to write about enchantment as something that is registered in the realm of magic/the magical and yet is embodied as a daily feminist practice.

Was it a mere coincidence that when I stayed at places where I was enchanted my back pain waned and my fatigue level was normal (as a sign that my Graves' disease was kept in check)? It would be, had there not been a strong pattern of a diminished feeling of pain when I was visiting specific sites and cities in Montenegro, Iceland, Spain, Ecuador, Austria, New Zealand, and Nepal, where I was intensely enchanted.[12] This is why I dare to play around with the idea that enchantment can function as an antidote to feeling pain.

According to political theorist and philosopher Jane Bennett, people can cultivate in themselves the ability to experience enchantment.[13] She points out that these moments of enchantment can "be cultivated and intensified by artful means," by mixing "artifice and spontaneity" and by practicing a stance of "generosity to the world."[14] Building on her suggestions, I highlight three practices that can simultaneously cultivate and signify moments of feminist enchantment. These three practices are forgetting/being spellbound, embodying the erotic as a life force, and being playful.

## 1. Forgetting, a.k.a. Being Spellbound

Watching the northern lights dance from inside a Buubble (transparent igloo/bubble) in Iceland was the only thing on my bucket list that year. Because Iceland was an expensive place to stay, Renzo and I were staying in the country for a total of four nights. You can imagine, then, that when I was able to snatch the last available spot at the Buubble on our last night in Iceland, I was beyond thrilled. As the stay at the Buubble was sold as part of a tour package, we spent most of the day being shuttled with four other people in a big van from one tourist site to another: Thingvellir National Park, Geyser Hot Spring, Gullfoss waterfall, and a secret lagoon, all of which were mesmerizing in their own ways. But I was so impatient to get to the igloos. Finally, around 10:00 p.m., we were dropped off at an undisclosed location where we saw the igloos at last. There was another group of six people who joined us there. We gathered in a small main lodge, where the only two bathrooms and showers were. After a short orientation, each couple was escorted to their igloo in a different spot on the property. The six igloos were all located within a short walking distance of the main lodge.

From our igloo, we could see the silhouette of nearby igloos. Since it was a transparent igloo, we could see everything outside (which was the point) and other people could see us inside our igloo, although the trees surrounding the igloo were supposed to give us a sense of privacy. I must admit it was an experience I could not quite grasp: it felt like being outside, but yet I was still inside. I was disoriented, but in a good, enchanted way. It truly felt as though I was in a movie of some sort. The igloo itself was shaped literally like a bubble, or a globe, except that its floor was flat and perched on a raised wooden deck. The igloo was quite spacious, especially compared to a regular camping tent. Inside, there was a cute setup of a comfortable bed with white furry pillows and a small rattanesque table with small lights and a small green plant for décor. Attached to the igloo was a short transparent tunnel, as a transition area. To go in and out of this bubble, I had to zip and unzip two doors, one at the end of the tunnel and another one for the igloo.

Because the tour company would pick all of us up at 8:00 a.m., we only had a relatively short period of time to stay in the bubble. I did want to see the northern lights, so I tried to stay awake all night. Renzo had asked me to wake him up if I saw the northern lights after he fell asleep. I was sitting in my bed, meditating with my mala bead, when around 2:30 a.m., I felt really cold. I woke Renzo up to ask him to go to the main lodge to figure out how to turn the heater back on. It was getting cold inside, and I could see some snow on top of the dome of our igloo, which impeded my vision of the night sky. Surely, I did not want to miss my chance of seeing the northern lights! When he came back from the main lodge, he told me to go outside.

"Is that the lights?" he asked while pointing up. The lights were not bright green like the pictures I often saw on the Internet. They were more white-blue-ish against the dark winter sky.

"I think so," I answered tentatively. I had never seen the northern lights before, so how could I be sure?

At first, the lights formed an arc, akin to that of a rainbow. Then, they started to move and dance. A few moments later, the lights were pouring down on us, like a powerful waterfall. I tried to sweep the night sky with my eyes, sparkling with the thrill. I felt my neck extending as far as it could go. I did not want to blink, as I was afraid I might miss some of its moves. The time, and we, stood still.

Neither of us let out a single word. We were simply spellbound. English professor Rita Felski has the perfect description of what it means to be enchanted that wholly captures my state of being in that moment: "an arresting of motion, a sense of being transfixed, spellbound, unable to move, even as your mind is transported elsewhere. . . . You are sucked in, swept up, spirited away, you feel yourself enfolded in a blissful embrace. You are mesmerized, hypnotized, possessed. You strain to reassert yourself, but finally you give in, you stop struggling, you yield without a murmur."[15] Being sucked into the mesmerizing motion of the light, I forgot that it had been a long day of sitting in the car that was not particularly friendly to my back pain. I even forgot the cold air of the night flicking my skin and my ears at thirty-four degrees Fahrenheit. I was, as Felski sums it up so accurately, "so entirely caught up in an aesthetic object that nothing else seems to matter."[16]

When we are enchanted, we are caught in the unexpected moments between the magical and the marvelous. We succumb to the grandeur that is being offered so generously in the moment. And in that moment, we somehow forget everything that is going on in our lives, including our body-in-pain. We are taken away into a world unto itself, "out of [our]selves" and "into an altered state of consciousness,"[17] where we have no control over our senses even as they operate "in high gear."[18] This feeling of being "oblivious to your surroundings, your past, your everyday life; you exist only in the present" gives way to a sense of "rapturous self-forgetting."[19] We may even "forget" the pain that we are feeling (even if only briefly, during those exact moments of enchantment).[20] Indeed, when we are fully immersed in enchantment—when our mind and inner critic do not run the show—the body is cued to shift, and we can start anew.[21]

This is why forgetting—being spellbound and transfixed—particularly during moments of enchantment, is crucial in shifting our pain because it crafts and charts a space where we can cultivate a new, different, and defiant way of perceiving our pain. Forgetting as a form of enchantment works to create a rupture that can disturb not only the narrative we may have of ourselves and our pain but also our routine and bodily memory, especially those that revolve around tending to our pain.

Forgetting and forgetfulness, rather than being considered as flaws, can be framed as feminist and subversive as they allow us to forget to carry pain in "the normal and the ordinary" way.[22] They invite us to find an "alternative mode of knowing" our pain.[23] Thus, to forget as a form of feminist enchantment is to forget how one *ought* to carry one's pain and to refuse to suffer in the manner that we are taught to suffer and have experienced suffering. It is to forget how we are supposed to live our lives (e.g., that we are to prioritize work and save up for retirement) and to forget that we are supposed to feel guilty when not being productive. Instead, to make time for enchantment is to take back and claim ownership of our time—how we structure and spend our time. It is to prioritize doing things that we enjoy and going to places that can take us to those moments of enchantment.

To forget, then, is to consider anew the pain that is being felt. The moment when we experience feminist enchantment is therefore important because it can expose us to the strangeness of pain. It can make our pain feel foreign to us. It can turn even our most chronic and faithful pain into a stranger. And in rendering pain as a stranger, it opens up a possibility for us to learn new ways of getting to know and carrying the pain. Perhaps what we need to let go of is not necessarily the pain itself but the fear of getting to know pain better.

## 2. Embodying the Erotic

Living in Hawai'i, I have snorkeled quite a bit. But snorkeling with playful sea lions in the Galápagos? That was a first. The snorkeling was part of an eight-day cruise on a sixteen-passenger maximum catamaran. (When I was not on the boat and feeling like I was about to die from the most horrible sea sickness I have ever experienced in my life, I actually had the best, most enchanting time of my life!) The cruise took me to several islands in the Galápagos: South Plaza, Santa Fe, Floreana, Santa Cruz, Isabela, and Fernandina. Sea lions certainly were not the only creatures I was captivated by. I was endearingly charmed by the blue-footed boobies (even when they were not doing the mating dance that I had watched on YouTube), Galápagos penguins, and lava herons, as I kayaked along the shoreline of Champion Islet. Throughout the various excursions, I also saw hundreds of iguanas piling on top of each other, one of the oldest tortoises mating and making (what I would identify as) grunting noises, and a crab nibbling on a dead rat, which was more than I had expected to see.

But in that moment of observing, forgetting, being mesmerized by the sea lion colonies that swam freely as they glided in the water with ease, and being aware that I was in the water with them, and being in such close proximity to them, I felt energized. A surge of vitality electrified my entire body. I was smiling from the core of my being. I suppose if a wound, to loosely paraphrase Rumi, is the crack where the light enters, my entire body must have been pores of the wound, as I felt the light blasting through my existence through these fissures. I felt uninhibitedly full. Indeed, enchantment is often described as a "mood of fullness, plenitude, or liveliness, a sense of having had one's nerves or circulation or concentration powers tuned up or recharged."[24] In that exact moment, I sure was recharged, my body tingling with energy. I was flowing and overflowing. I could not tell where my existence ended and the other began. As Zen Buddhist priest, author, and artist Zenju Earthlynn Manuel observes of her own experience, "Enchantment is to sense myself without boundaries."[25] At that moment, I felt boundless: the cool ocean water became me, and I became one with and part of nature.

This fullness felt during enchantment can be quite powerful and subversive if we reconfigure its meaning to be a moment of reembodying the power of the erotic. Certainly, the erotic here is not to be understood solely in its limited sexual sense but rather in Black feminist thinker Audre Lorde's sense of the word, as "an assertion of the life force of women."[26] The erotic, Lorde writes, "is an internal sense of satisfaction to which, once we have experienced it, we know we can aspire. For having experienced the fullness of this depth of feeling and recognizing its power, in honor and self-respect we can require no less of ourselves." In this sense, the erotic registers in the same plane as the experience of enchantment in that it shares the feeling of internal satisfaction and tells us "which of our various life endeavors bring us closest to that fullness."[27]

By way of Lorde's different iterations of the erotic, all of which use the word "full," I want to wholly embrace the meaning of the erotic that is about feeling full from the inside.

When the erotic provides us with information about which activity brings us to a feeling of fullness, it functions as a compass that leads us to our very own antidote to pain. That is, if pain is a disorienting tool that pushes us away from something, the erotic can become our orienting tool that leads us toward something. In this way, the erotic can work as an "episteme, a critical mode through which we may attain excellence."[28] This means that to embody the erotic we need to return to the body as a system of knowing. We need to rely on our own bodily senses and feelings, and be aware of and embrace that feeling of fullness when it is felt, and refuse to live otherwise.[29]

The power of the erotic can also help us reconnect with our body and ourselves.[30] From a phenomenological perspective, pain and suffering produce alienation from one's own body and identity, as well as from one's own sense of self and being. Suffering makes us feel as if we are not at home in our own body.[31] Of course, not all suffering "is alienating."[32] However, as philosopher Fredrik Svenaeus points out, pain often alienates us from our own bodies, as well as "from the world we live in by making it an unhomelike place to be. . . . This is so because the body in pain forces the person to focus her attention on it, instead of on the meaning structures of the world she is normally engaged in. Chronic pain makes life poor and enforces isolation."[33] This "double alienation" of pain often makes me feel not only that my body betrays me but also that my body is "not me" or mine.[34] I do not recognize it; I do not know how it works or what it wants. I do not know how to connect with it, despite countless hours trying to communicate with it.

For instance, avoiding all inflammatory food and doing the exercise that my doctor recommended usually helped with my Graves' disease. However, at times, even as I obey the doctor, my thyroid test levels come back abnormal. When that happens, I feel that my body is a stranger to me, or I to it. In this way, pain becomes "a distancing phenomenon."[35]

It distances oneself from one's body, as well as from others and other bodies. Indeed, when I am in pain, all I want to or can do is to cower in bed and stay away from people. At its excruciating worst, my pain makes me want to distance myself from my own body, to leave all of its painful glory, to leave this world.

Enchantment, however, dispels this alienation and reconnects a person to their own mind/body/spirit/self/surroundings. When I was standing at the edge of a cliff in Galápagos, marveling at the Darwin Lake down below and breathing in the crisp, fresh air that filled me up from the inside, I felt as though the elixir of the erotic as a life force was being injected into my body. (This reminds me of Bennett's point that we should "pursue a life with *moments* of enchantment rather than an enchanted way of life.")[36] What enchantment does to me is, as scholars Ann Burlein and Jackie Orr articulate so beautifully, that it "activates sensual matters in uncertain ways, via rhythm, play, poetic gesture, vibratory frequencies that confuse or re-fuse familiar temporalities, and initiate transformed perception."[37] When the sensual part of me was activated, not only did I feel alive but I also felt empowered. I was reclaiming my body and giving it permission to feel all there was to feel, to be reconnected to all my relations and sensations. When I am living in that moment of enchantment, I know that my pain is still there, but how I perceive it, how I carry it, has shifted. It is as if I can tell my pain to sit still and wait patiently for me, while I enjoy the mesmerizing beauty, and it listens to me. Here, I imagine enchantment as that moment when pain is in alignment with life.

To feel thoroughly enchanted when we have been told to simply live with, suppress, or avoid the pain can be subversive. For once we know what being enchanted and embodying the power of the erotic feels like, we will no longer allow our life to be wilted or wasted. In Lorde's words, "For as we begin to recognize our deepest feelings, we begin to give up, of necessity, being satisfied with suffering and self-negation, and with the numbness which so often seems like their only alternative in our society. Our acts against oppression become integral with self, motivated and empowered from within. In touch with the erotic, I become less willing to accept powerlessness, or those other supplied states of being which are not native to me, such as resignation, despair, self-effacement, depression, self-denial."[38] It is in this sense of the erotic as a means to refuse to be powerless or to succumb to pain that I claim that enchantment works as a subversive feminist embodied daily practice. When we embrace the erotic and feel enchanted, we are less willing to endure suffering. The erotic distances us from the willingness to cast ourselves as sufferers. The erotic *moment* of enchantment is the permission slip that allows us to take a break from our pain, especially pain that is caused by patriarchy and other forms of structural inequality, and to take back that feeling of being alive, connected (rather than alienated), and powerful.

### 3. Bodily Remembering, a.k.a. Being Playful

"Oh. My. Heavens! *I am here! I am heeeeeere!!!!*" I was screaming on the inside when I reached Barcelona. I stood in front of a magical place, Casa Batlló. It was a tall building; counting its windows vertically, I was guessing it had six floors. Parts of it looked as though it was made from giant skeletons; parts of it looked as though it was a whimsical fairyland filled with bright colors in different shades of blue, green, pink, and yellow—something we would see at a magical rainbow unicorn theme park, if there is one. A spiritual melancholy in the shape of a cross was pointing out of its roof. It was truly an enchanting site to behold.

The sections of the house that were open to the public were restored to provide us with a glimpse of its original beauty. I walked up the staircase with its curvy railing and on to the living room. From the audio and virtual guide screen, I could see how the living room appeared many, many decades ago. The playful shapes of every single thing in that house would be tantalizing even to the most unartistic of eyes. Where I would usually find edges, there were none. How could a person come up with such ideas? I wanted to have that kind of creativity.

I spent the next two days visiting Antoni Gaudí's other masterpieces, wanting to dive deeper inside his brilliant mind. From Park Güell, I learned about his humility and failure. He was commissioned to establish an exclusive community of mansions that would have splendid architectural designs everywhere your eyes turned, with spectacular views of the city. But the vision never really materialized. He only completed two houses. No one wanted to live more than an hour from the city by horse carriage. So even a genius suffered setbacks and failures.

La Sagrada Familia, the famous church, made me realize that the human brain was capable of so much more and then some. At least Gaudí's brain was. It was ten o'clock in the morning when I entered one of the two church towers. I chose the passion façade because I liked the sound of it. In Spain, tickets are generally timed, and you have to show up before your time or lose your spot. This practice is harsh but fair. It regulates the number of people visiting at a specific time and protects these heritage sites. It forced me to plan ahead.

The steps to the tower were steep. I could feel my skin drenched by the sun's heat, the hot sweat sticking to my shirt. How I longed for a cold, refreshing shower! Once I reached the top, I could see the view and some of the roof's meticulous artwork. "From above" is my favorite kind of view: the surrounding roofs and roads made for an intricate and intriguing maze. Things do indeed appear more beautiful and meaningful from above.

Many parts of the church were still under construction, and cranes and fences marred the view. But to me they were a reminder that human beings are never able to complete all of what we set out to do in this world. No matter how productive we are, how hard we work during our lifetime, how fully we have lived our lives, when we die, there will still be projects left unfinished, and places not yet explored. The self will never be complete. As productive as Gaudí was, he left this world not having completed his grand church. Gazing at the unfinished masterpiece, I felt freed by that realization. I no longer felt the urgency to complete everything, and to complete everything *now*. What pressure that was!

If George Levine in his book *Darwin Loves You: Natural Selection and the Re-Enchantment of the World* says that Charles Darwin's world is an enchanted one—in a "nontheistic" way in that it turns to nature instead of "to supernaturalist religion" as an alternative source of enchantment—then I would say that Gaudí's world is also an enchanted one.[39] In this case, enchantment does not come from nature but from art, artifact, and architecture. This was evident when I was walking inside the church. The left side of the church's glass windows had different colors from the right, to showcase the changing colors of the sun from when it is rising to when it is setting. The left side had brighter colors like red, orange, and yellow—because the morning sun shone through those windows—and the right side had different shades of blue and green, for the cool afternoon sun. That morning the sun was as bright as it could ever be and it lit up the walls and floors of the church in playful, vibrant colors. It made walking inside the church feel like walking in an enchanted forest with delightful, super-bright colors that were blinding to the eyes. I stood there, in awe, in love, in gratitude, with all kinds of mixed feelings. In that moment, I felt a childlike excitement about life, about magic, about a magical life. This echoes Bennett's sentiment that "the overall effect of enchantment is . . . a fleeting return to childlike excitement about life."[40]

He might have been brilliant and devoted to his God, but most of all, Gaudí was playful. From his architectural legacies, I would read him as being a child at heart and a believer in the wondrous magic of play. That was what I perceived was alive in him and, as I stood there, I realized that that had been dying in me. He allowed playfulness and magic to guide his life, his creation, his architecture. And he was celebrated for being playful, for being different. His brilliance comes from his playfulness. I wonder what kind of society we would create, what kind of person I would end up becoming, if we did not ask adults to repress their urge to play with everything, even in their jobs. What would our world (metaphorically and literally—the physical landscape within which we exist) be like if play is part of work, of life itself?

I agree with Bennett, who mentions that play is a strategy to foster enchantment.[41] To feel more moments of enchantment, we need to play and be more playful. Traveling can be considered a form of play as it encourages people to play with their identity and ways of being and living in this world. Playfulness during travel can be understood as "an openness to being a fool, which is a combination of not worrying about competence, not being self-important, not taking norms as sacred, and finding ambiguity and double edges a source of wisdom and delight."[42] This state of being open to being a fool allows us to shift the power dynamic when encountering others: we become filled with curiosity, creativity, and childlike wonder. We genuinely seek to know: *How can we play with others and even with our pain? How do we meet our pain at the point of play? What does it mean and what will happen to us when we do not believe anymore in the story that pain has been telling us as "truth," but rather see it as a lighthearted fiction and tale?* Thus, to be playful means that we embrace the excitement of the unknown and the not knowing. We have an open-hearted willingness, a genuine curiosity, to be entertained by what may come, even if it forces us to see our insignificance and ignorance.[43] Moreover, to return to a playful way of being is to return to our body's natural state—indeed, "culture itself is formed at its deepest level by the ludic or 'play-element.'"[44]

Enchantment provides us with a safe space, an affective boundary, where we do not have to believe (i.e., we can forget) the story that pain has been telling us, or what others have been telling us pain means. And instead, we can begin to create playful ways to experience and carry pain. To be enchanted, then, we must have the ability to play with the self, spirit, and other, and the ability to be playful and be engaged in the playfulness of self/other. Being playful becomes our daily and embodied mode of engaging with ourselves, our pain, and other humans, as well as other nonhuman and nonliving entities.

As a final note to this section on feminist enchantment, I want to make clear that if I insist in proposing a new concept that I call "feminist enchantment," it is because I want to have a language to name that spe-

cific moment when pain still exists, yet its existence is rendered meaningless, drowned out by the magic that lights up the brain in different,
enchanting, and empowering ways—the moment when I dare to reclaim
my body, my power, and my agency.[45]

## Traveling with a Twist: From Repetition to New Habitual Body Practice

Travel writings are replete with stories of healing. In 1875, for instance,
Isabella Bird, a British "Lady Traveler" and writer, published her book,
*The Hawaiian Archipelago: Six Months among the Palm Groves, Coral
Reefs, and Volcanoes of the Sandwich Islands*. She described traveling to
Hawai'i as healing the symptoms of the illness she had suffered. Her
improved health, she believed, was partly due to the "enchanted" "fairy
land" and "isolated" areas of Hawai'i.[46]

People have indeed traveled to different places in pursuit of a healthy
body.[47] Narratives that travel can improve health have been around
since ancient times.[48] In more modern times, travel has been "prescribed" to cure illness and framed as "a diversion" for people who have
depression or other emotional issues.[49] Many women travel writers cite
travel as the "miraculous" cure for their emotional and physical illnesses.[50] Popular books such as *Eat, Pray, Love: One Woman's Search
for Everything across Italy, India, and Indonesia* and *Wild: From Lost to
Found on the Pacific Crest Trail* do indeed tell stories of how pain propels women to travel to heal.

I want to propose here that it is not travel per se that is healing but
the *new* habitual body that is created during travel that may lead to healing. Traveling does not automatically produce a new habitual body or
allow us to meet our stranger-selves, of course. If we travel abroad only
to recreate routines we had at home, we may not shift our relationship
with our body or pain.

When we travel, we have an opportunity to create new habits. Traveling produces distance that is important in making space for us to

practice enchantment that can "erase the pain of existence in one world by escaping to another, where one lives in an enchanted state of non-identity, where one is free to be another and see one's self as another."[51] Traveling also creates opportunities for new experiences that call forth new dimensions of ourselves. Indeed, this may be why some people travel when they say they want to "find" themselves: they want to summon a different aspect of themselves that they may not even know exists or have never met before. They want to give birth to that part of the self that is still snuggled comfortably inside their (metaphorical) womb.[52] By traveling, they hope to find "the strangeness in themselves" or, at least, to become a stranger to their own "country, language, sex, and identity" and, I would even argue, pain.[53] As English professor Joyce Kelley lays out, "When that body goes abroad, the mind is 'moved' by foreign sights, and the body moves away from its everyday habits. In travel, the usual becomes unusual, and even small changes in routine can call for large adjustments."[54] During travels, we often feel that our body is being "displaced" and therefore "foreign and thus new."[55] This newness is what may elicit the creation of a new habitual body and an enchanting experience, although not always. In this section, I am thus intrigued not by spontaneous moments of enchantment (as discussed in the previous section) but by ways of doing things—in my specific case, walking—that function as a repetition but with a twist, and still lead to enchantment (i.e., forgetting, embodying the erotic, and being playful) *and* the formation of a new habitual body.

## From Walking to In-Habit-ing a New Body

I visited Kotor, Montenegro, in August 2017. The visuality of the city delivered its promise: the emerald green color of Kotor Bay against the backdrop of the mountains, covered with many different shades of green, melted something inside me. The energy of any place could never really come through an image, so I was pleased to learn that Kotor was not only as beautiful as its representations on social media (if not more beautiful) but also had the kind of aura that enchanted me.

I stayed in Kotor for two weeks, at a small studio apartment in old town, inside the fortress. My apartment was on the third floor; most first floors of the old buildings in the fortress have been turned into shops or restaurants. Buildings inside the fortress had gray- and beige- (greige-?) colored bricks on most of their walls. The alleys were small and intimate, and there being a pedestrian-only zone adds to the sense of closeness and coziness of the place. Luckily, my apartment was only a few steps away from the South Gate, through which I could easily access the main street and therefore buses, a farmers'/open market, and a path to Kotor Bay. Everything I needed was within a short walk, so walking became my habit.

My daily routine in Kotor went something like this: I would wake up usually around 6:00 or 7:00 in the morning. I would write for two hours. Then, on some mornings, and definitely on Saturdays because they had more selection, I would go to the farmers' market, which was right outside the fortress, a five-minute walk. The market was open from 7:00 until early afternoon, around 2:00. I would usually spend about five euros for fruits, four euros for vegetables, and two euros for olives. This supply would last about two to three days. The fruit I bought at the market was the highlight of my trip. Peaches were especially sweet and fragrant. They were deliciously ripe. The feeling of biting into something that was perfectly soft with oozing juices allowed me to embody the erotic Lorde describes. These fresh fruits made my body feel alive, as if their nectars were the magical elixir that revitalized my body, made me forget my chronic pain and instead remember how my body would naturally feel—vibrant, light, and playful. Sometimes I got a high-energy boost, so much so that I felt like dancing and being playful, just from biting into these fruits!

Being able to eat affordable, easily accessible, and fresh fruits (no need to stock up since I could always walk for five minutes to get them) made it easier for me to keep my chronic illness under control. To reduce inflammation, I have to avoid coffee, soy, eggs, wheat, dairy, cheese, corn, canola oil, and pork. The availability and affordability of fresh fruits and vegetables at the market helped calm my chronic illnesses. (In Honolulu, where organic fruits were more expensive and less juicy than in Kotor, and I had to drive usually once a week to the grocery/market to get them, it was harder for me to stay on this healthy diet.) After going to the market, I would then walk home, have my breakfast, take a shower, and go back to writing, until lunchtime. After lunch, I would explore the city either by bus, on foot, or in an organized tour, and return home at night, having dinner at one of the nearby restaurants or at home.

Perhaps a digression is necessary here, if only to clarify how the materiality of the city where I was able to enjoy affordable fresh fruits and walk places is revealing of my class privilege in a transnational context.[56] (This is to say that living and working in the United States, I benefit from the imperial power of America.) In the United States, I was an associate professor at a state university, earning a decent salary, enough to get by in one of the most expensive cities in the United States. But in Kotor (or many places I traveled to during my sabbatical year), it was possible and affordable for me, with my American salary, to rent a place in a relatively expensive part of Kotor, the old town, that enabled me to walk and enjoy fresh fruits easily. But my lodgings, which cost me 52 USD/night, might not be as affordable for many people who live and work there; their national minimum wage in 2017 was 325 USD per month.[57] Not only in Montenegro but also in the United States, we often find this inequality. Sociologist Tanya Golash-Boza writes that in the United States, people of African descent and/or who came from Latin American countries often live where it is harder to buy fresh produce or healthy foods.[58] These places usually do not have parks or jogging trails, and instead, are environmentally toxic. This is why the subject of health and well-being can never be divorced from structural issues. (More on this in chapter 6.)

To return us to my discussion of my daily life in Kotor: I noticed that after the first full day of walking, my back pain worsened. I decided to change my shoes from tennis shoes to a pair of walking sandals, but it helped only a tiny bit. Gradually, after the first week, I noticed a change in my body, or rather, in how I felt my body. I felt lighter. Soon after, I almost forgot that I had back pain. The moment I realized that, I tried to pinpoint the magical variable. Was it the bed? The bed in my studio apartment was rock hard. I then remembered that a long time earlier, a few people had suggested that I sleep on the floor to help with my back pain. I tried it once or a couple of times back then, but it did not help. But experiencing this release from my back pain, I wondered if they might have been right: could sleeping on a hard surface help my back? But when I was in Madrid, a couple of months after my visit to Kotor, the bed was soft, or rather, lumpy, and my back was fine then, too. I concluded that it could not have been just the bed.

I suspected that this might have a lot to do with walking as a form of enchantment, a repetition with a twist. When I was at home in Honolulu, I would drive to get to places. Driving, flying, or biking inevitably affects how we orient ourselves in space, how we experience our travels, and how we encounter others.[59] Walking affected how I experienced my body and what I was able to perceive with my body. When walking, I used different muscles. Walking itself became an exercise that I enjoyed. Because walking is registered at a different tempo than driving, it contributes to how I experience enchantment—we can slow down or speed up our pace to cultivate enchantment.[60] In my particular case, walking allowed me to experience more moments of enchantment because it slowed down the usual tempo of how I encountered the world. It allowed me to stop, smell, and sense at any time, and make decisions based on this perception.

When I was walking, I let my body lead me. This is a different practice from the neoliberal exercise of walking to meet the goal of having a certain number of steps per day and obsessively checking the Fitbit, which records (and performs surveillance on) the movement of the body. I let my body, instead of the goal or the gadget, lead me. This means that I would walk aimlessly inside the fortress in Kotor, stopping at different stores, checking out souvenirs, or sitting inside an old church and absorbing its peaceful energy as my body wanted it. Even though I carried a map of the fortress with me, I did not use it. Instead, my body oriented me to the environment and took whatever turns it wanted. I had no specific place that I needed to be. I would feel with my body where I would want to stop for dinner, my sense of smell alerting me to what was cooking at the moment. I did not rely on Yelp or other people's reviews to guide me. This practice became a form of connecting with my body (relying on it as a system of knowing) and of being playful in going about my day (and my meals). I would ask myself, *What does my body want to do/eat right now?*

At other times, I would decide where to eat on the basis of the location. For instance, one evening, I passed a square that was facing a church, with a violinist playing a beautiful song. The food at the restaurant with open-air seating facing the square was not amazing, but the ambiance was beyond serene. Letting my body make these decisions, I often found myself being satisfied with whatever was served. This daily satisfaction, contentment, and pleasure that were body based and relied on the power of the erotic allowed me to be enchanted, moment by moment. Walking does wonders for my body!

Another place where I cultivated walking as part of my feminist enchantment practice and new habitual body was Madrid, which I visited in October 2017. Being there made me feel as though I was emerging from a spa with a sense of freshness, of being completely relaxed and rejuvenated. My skin was tingling with the freshness of blood flowing. My lips were offering smiles to strangers, dogs, delivery trucks—everything. I felt like a fully charged phone.

For me, this feeling of being enchanted in Madrid was also related to walking as part of my feminist enchantment practice that I repeated every day, but with a twist. This means that my practice was not just about walking every day but also a matter of *where* (the different places) I walked to, and what I experienced there, even when I went to the same place, that contributed to my experiencing enchantment. How could I not be enchanted when every morning I walked to Chocolatería San Ginés to get some *churros* and a cup of hot chocolate? Their *churros* were thin and long, unlike most *churros* I had eaten in the United States. The consistency was also different. Theirs were softer yet crispier (you have to try it to believe it!) and tasted more buttery. When dipped in their perfectly thick (but not clumpy) hot chocolate, they tasted even better. (Any culture that allows me to dip my breakfast in hot chocolate is the kind of culture I would worship.)

Savoring the softness of the crispy *churros* and the sweetness of the hot chocolate mixed delicately in my mouth, I would instantly feel infused by the power of the erotic. It was as if I was taking a one-way express train to Foodgasmville, a.k.a. heaven. In fact, if heaven had an address, it would surely be where Chocolatería San Ginés stood, all three of them. Believe it or not, they actually had three shops adjacent to each other; the one in the middle was open twenty-four hours a day, and usually had a long line. That was actually how I found the place: I was walking a few short minutes away from my hotel—a two-star hotel right in the city center, which had a bathroom so small I could not even spread my arms in it—when I saw people lining up outside the shop. Naturally, out of curiosity, I had to join the queue and try it for myself.

(Speaking of the hotel, although this has no relevance to the story I am telling, I have to share that during my check-in at the hotel in Madrid, the two Filipina women who worked as cleaners were summoned by the receptionist to do the important work of translation without being paid. I could not speak Spanish; the receptionist could not speak English. These women's work exemplifies one of the many unpaid tasks that women of color across the globe are being asked to do to support the global tourism industry. I was a woman of color, too, but in that moment, I was playing the role of the ugly tourist who could not speak the local language, and hence was complicit in benefiting from other women of color's unpaid work. Recognizing the awkwardness of the situation, the Filipina women and I exchanged smiles—the kind that could only be decoded through the way we filled meanings through our eyes, through how we looked at each other, the kind that acknowledged the irony of how we, three South-east Asian women who looked more alike to each other than not, were standing literally on the opposite sides of the desk, speaking not in our native languages and not to connect with one another but in a language foreign to us and to help the white man do his job.)

From my hotel, I also enjoyed walking to the fresh market. Mercado de San Miguel was where I spent some of my lunchtimes. The abundance of food—of *tapas*, of mozzarella, of olives neatly arranged on skewers, mixed with different assortments of cheeses, pickled onions, and anchovies—was a visual feast for my hungry eyes. I could even smell fresh fruit as soon as I walked inside. Their natural scent was like an aphrodisiac that made me feel alive—once again embodying the erotic moment of enchantment.

Then, there were parks that I walked to every single day for the six days I was there. And this was not because I ran out of things to do. Retiro Park was in some ways like Central Park in New York City. It was massive in size. Central Park is bigger, with 843 acres, compared to Retiro Park's 350. But still. Located in the city, Retiro Park was full of fountains, gorgeous sculptures, blossoming colorful flowers, and lovely ponds. There was a pond in front of the Crystal Palace where I would sit, looking at the ducks and black swans swimming calmly and the birds chirping away. I remember sitting there thinking, *Would this be what the Garden of Eden looked like?* The glow of the sun reflected on the water, shimmering gold with diamond sparkles. Some children fed the ducks. I watched them interact, their hands reaching out, waiting for the ducks to take some food. They smiled with so much joy. My heart smiled with them. I melted into liquid nonexistence. There, but not there. Feeling, but not riding the emotions.

When I traveled to Madrid again in the spring—I loved Madrid so much that I went there twice during my sabbatical year—the pond did not feel as magical or charming/calming. But I found the different colors of roses at La Rosaleda garden at the back end of Retiro Park magnificent. I walked there every single day. One afternoon I sat in the rose garden for two hours, and by chance, I witnessed a couple getting engaged. The man brought a group of violinists to serenade the proposal. It was an enchanting performance of beautiful music, the fragrant smell and vibrant color of the roses, and the blossoming love. It made me fall in love, too, with life.

It also matters not only that I can walk places but that I can walk places at night, alone. When I was in Kotor and Madrid, I stayed at places that allowed me to roam at night and feel safe. I noticed the different sensations my body was feeling when walking at night, as opposed to during the day. In Madrid, I walked to Plaza de Oriente, a nineteenth-century park right outside the Royal Palace of Madrid. I visited it every evening, around 11:00 after dinner—restaurants usually opened for dinner around 9:00. I would sit on the bench close to Teatro Real and a row of nice restaurants, facing the fountain. I loved hearing the cling-clang of spoons, glasses, and plates as they met and greeted each other, the buzzing sound of people conversing in languages I did not understand but could feel. My chest became full seeing couples hugging, kissing, and touching each other on the long white bench on the far left side of the park, Jardines de Lepanto, where it was dark. Different couples would sit on the bench each night, but they would do similar things. Loving on each other. At the same park, I would also enjoy observing people walking their dogs slowly, leisurely. Sitting in the park at night was my lullaby, and it delivered me to soothing sleepiness. Walking alone at night created a different sensation in my body, akin to taking a hot bath at night or quietly savoring a glass of pinot noir. Marvelously soothing.

Being able to walk at night matters because in both of these places, I was a woman traveling alone. Where and when a woman, cis- or trans-, can walk alone is often limited by the likelihood of her being harassed. If I had stayed at a different place where it might not have been safe for women to walk alone at night, I might not have been able to experience these enchanting moments.[61]

*Repetition and the New Habitual Body*

In proposing that walking produces a new habitual body and allows me to experience enchantment, I want to emphasize the notion of enchantment as a "practice." As a bodily practice, enchantment requires repetition. This notion of enchantment as repetition can be found in the meaning of the word itself: the word "enchant" can be traced to the French word "*chanter*," which means "to sing."[62] The *enchant*ment in a song can be found in its refrain, which serves a "catalytic function" that can transform "sense" into "nonsense and then a new sense of things" by way of "the repetition of word sounds" that "exaggerates the tempo of an ordinary phrase" and "renders a meaningful phrase nonsense."[63] In other words, that very repetition, when coupled with the manipulation of the tempo, can evoke a sense of enchantment.

What is important to note about repetition in enchantment is that it takes the form of a "spiral repetition" where "things repeat but with a twist. And this twist—or to use the Lucretian term, *swerve*—makes possible new formations."[64] This means that it is not that I create a new habitual body solely by repeating my walk but that my walk, which I do every day, brings me a different "twist" of experience each day. Repeating with a twist can also be understood as repetition working "'intensively' . . . taking the singular object of one's attention to what Deleuze calls the *n*th power."[65] That is, the more I practice my walk, the more intensified is the experience of walking itself for me, which can then lead to transformation. Bennett points it out best: "That which repeats itself also transforms itself. Because each iteration occurs in a . . . unique context, each turn of the spiral enters into a new and distinctive assemblage."[66] Repetition that enchants need not be intentional but "can be singular 'disparates' that connect, combine, and differentiate in multiple ways."[67] In my daily walk, even as I went to the same Retiro Park, I would stumble upon and pay attention to different sites and objects. One day, I was enchanted by the ducks, other days by its rose garden.

This daily walking, the repetition with a twist, not only enchants but it also creates a new habitual body. Habits have indeed been *"performed in and by our bodies"* and in turn re/make who we are.[68] This creation of a new habitual body matters because as we create a new habitual body, we may be "practicing a new body, one which does not include pain."[69] Thus, when I keep practicing my walk, I not only cultivate "an eye for the wonderful" but also, I improve my ability to be enchanted by what the twist brings me.[70] It is an exercise of both detoxifying the gaze and recycling awe.

The key here, according to Bennett, is that the repetitions need to be "distinctive enough to cause wonder, to jar from the usual ruts of experience. Another way of putting this point is to say that the beautiful thing's form must provoke the experience of a gap between its form and our (default) sensibility. Without this gap—the space of perplexity, surprise, or confoundment—a beautiful thing will lack the considerable power required to immobilize limbs and animate objects."[71] Enchantment thus cannot happen when there is no element of "unpredictability" or the "mysterious."[72] Walking in new places I visited while traveling and repeating my walks with a twist provided me with that gap, between my default senses and the new experiences. In other words, the new environment, or the new way of experiencing the same environment, could then provoke the transformation of the "ecology of the self."[73] As I practiced this enchantment daily, the new habitual body, one that had a new relationship with pain, was gradually formed.

For readers who may wonder how the new habitual body differs from the concept of "habitus" that sociologist Pierre Bourdieu speaks of, please allow me to clarify briefly here. The creation of a new habitual body and the formation of habitus may be similar—both are produced by way of repetition performed by the body, and in both concepts, the body becomes a site upon which to inscribe social and class status. The new habitual body, however, is meant to disrupt the habitus. If the production of the body in the habitus relies more on subconscious learning, in the new habitual body, the body is freed from learning. The body is not taught to walk a certain way or at certain places to produce the classed/gendered/racialized body. The opposite happens: the new habitual body is produced by way of trusting the body and letting it be completely free (e.g., to go where it wants at that moment) and letting it create new habits, ones that can reset the body to carry pain differently. If habitus relies on structure,[74] the new habitual body frees the body from the structure. If habitus produces a certain kind of lifestyle,[75] the new habitual body is about constantly creating a twist even as we repeat—a nonlifestyle.

What I hope to make clear here is this: it is not traveling or walking per se that allows me to be enchanted and shift how I carry pain in my body. Of course, the act of walking itself is a good form of exercise that contributes to the overall well-being of my body. But if walking is not repeated with a playful twist that creates a jarring gap, it will not yield moments of enchantment.

When we experience moments of enchantment every day, that is when the new habitual body is produced. The new habitual body is produced out of experiencing enchantment every day—enchantment as an embodied practice—not merely out of walking per se. Thus, the new habitual body can be understood as a new mode of embodying the body that has a different relationship to pain, and deems enchantment as constitutive of its materiality/reality. It is important, therefore, that I clarify here that the feminist enchantment that I propose is *not* the kind of enchantment that the tourism industry offers us: going to a list of "enchanting" places, being herded from one place to another. That kind of experience is more exhausting than enchanting, at least for me.

## Conclusion

Chronic pain is only felt when it makes itself present to me, which then makes me remember that I have it. Practicing feminist enchantment allows me to forget my chronic illnesses, to push them to the background of my life. Hence, the discussion in this chapter similarly reflects that: chronic illness appears only in the "background" of the chapter, but not as I was detailing the moments (and concept) of feminist enchantment. When I was enchanted, the chronic pain simply was "forgotten"—that is indeed the point of this chapter.

Enchantment exists in the magical and marvelous spaces between the affective of the body and the imaginative of the mind. So magnificent is enchantment as an antidote to pain that I invite the readers to practice it in their everyday lives. By forgetting what we are supposed to remember about how to carry pain; by feeling full (embodying the erotic) even though we (especially as women of color) are constantly told to starve ourselves—physically, emotionally, financially, etc.; and by being playful even when we are taught that we need to act serious to be taken seriously, we can set ourselves up to experience moments of feminist enchantment. When embodied, feminist enchantment will reset our relationship with pain, with ourselves and our surrounding, and with how we live our lives.

It is true that traveling, especially abroad, can push us toward a path of enchantment, although there is no guarantee in that. Foreign environments can incite our body to play around with new practices. When we repeat these bodily practices with a twist, we intensify our chances of being enchanted and of creating a new habitual body. This new habitual body is the body that has shifted and uplifted (the context of) pain carried chronically by the body.

I want to remind the readers that although a foreign environment makes it easier for us to adopt new practices, that is not always the case. Some people travel abroad only to duplicate the practices they do at home (eat the same food, speak the same language). On the contrary, it is possible to stay at home and explore our surroundings differently so we can adopt a new habitual body nonetheless (e.g., we can explore different routes or pay attention to different things when walking to our workplace; we can slow down our walk; we can go to local events that remind our body to be playful; we can explore local museums and parks with childlike curiosity; we can kayak or hike at different nature sites; we can pretend to be a stranger to our own city; we can try a new recipe or buy a different jar of ready-made pomodoro sauce to spice up the spaghetti dinner we have every night, etc.).

Feminist enchantment can thus be practiced anywhere, not only in foreign environments. The most important thing about practicing feminist enchantment is to really listen to the body in order to know what it desires, what it wants to do, enjoy, eat, or where it wants to go at that particular moment. Of course, we cannot always do what it wants all the time. We do have to go to work even when our body wants to play with dolphins all day! But if we keep denying what the body wants (including during the weekends), then do not be surprised when soon enough, we will be disconnected from our body, and our pain will feel more intense.

Pain is a way for the body to speak to us, to let us know that something needs changing. Cultivating feminist enchantment as an embodied daily practice is a way to speak back to pain, to let it know that we are listening and making changes. It is also to be more aware of the connections that our mind/body has with its surroundings.

To end this chapter, I want to leave the readers with this simple question: What one thing can we do today to forget/be spellbound, embody the erotic, and be more playful—that is, to practice feminist enchantment, so that we can carry pain differently in our lives?

6

## How Does Where I Live Matter to My Pain?

I love traveling. Even when it leaves my anxiety bare, exposed to the callous touch of strangers. Even with all the grief that comes from brief interactions with unnamed border patrol officers, police officers, or shopkeepers. Even then. Like that one time in Germany, when I was driving and got pulled over by a cop who asked me for my passport when I had not done anything wrong. Or that time in Japan, when I was followed around by a shopkeeper who was afraid that I might steal something from them. Such is the rhythm of traveling while being a woman of color.

When harassment and discrimination frequently accompany my travels, kindness (even indifference) often feels like a trespasser. It makes me question all the possibilities of how it finds its way to where I am. *Can there be something that the governments do to provide their citizens with an environment where people are kinder and less likely to create pain in each other's lives, and instead, are more likely to carry their own and each other's pain in a more life-sustaining way?* My short visits to Iceland and New Zealand led me to a preliminary but hopeful answer: yes. Yes, there are programs and policies that governments can put in place to provide their citizens with access to well-being. In fact, no matter how radically we change our mind/perception, how hard we work with our body to process pain, and how diligently we practice feminist enchantment in our daily lives, if we do not have the structural support from our government, we will not be able to fully carry pain in a life-sustaining, humane, and feminist way. Sisyphus we will be. It is thus these programs and policies that prioritize the well-being of citizens, in what I call an "emotional contract," that will be the main focus of this chapter.

## My Travels to Iceland and New Zealand

I dug my spoon into a decent portion of rye bread ice cream, buried underneath a tall and decadent house-made whipped cream, drizzled with rhubarb syrup. I first saw it on Instagram. The minute I made it to Kaffi Loki in Reykjavik, Iceland, I had to have it. I let the sweet taste and sandy texture of the ice cream linger inside my mouth and took the extra time to savor it. It was surprisingly good. I say "surprisingly" because each time I had mentioned to anyone (friends or strangers) that I was planning to visit Iceland, they *all*, without exception, warned me that the food in Iceland was terrible *and* ridiculously expensive. "Be prepared to pay thirty dollars for an inedible burger!" a guy sharing a van to the airport in Nepal cautioned me.

But for the four nights Renzo and I visited Iceland, we were both happy with the food. Perhaps relying on our eyes and intuitions worked (we often subtly peeked through the windows to steal a glance at the food on the customers' plates before choosing a restaurant). Or, perhaps the couple of instances when we took time to go through online reviews paid off, too. Whatever way we ended up at these restaurants, we found the food, from eggs and herring to smoked trout and cottage cheese to mashed fish (*plokkfiskur*) and to beef in a pancake, to be exquisite. The price was not ridiculously expensive either. The rye bread ice cream, for instance, was 850 kr (5.90 USD), and the beef in a pancake that came with pickled onion, blue cheese, and hollandaise sauce was 1890 kr (13 USD). The price was comparable to that in the restaurants I frequented at home in the United States, and the payment process was convenient since all places I visited only took credit cards and did not accept cash.

When I asked what the local tipping rule was, one of the servers told me cheerfully, "We don't expect it. It's nice if you would like to leave a tip, but here, we are paid good wages so we don't rely on tips." Her response was a sweet sting to the American restaurant industry, which does not take care of its workers, who are paid inadequate wages and therefore have to rely on tips to supplement their income (an example of how structure—in this case, low wage—makes workers feel that they have to fend for themselves). Her emphasis on "we are paid good wages" also hinted at her seeming contentment at being supported by her employer through the good wage that she received. In other words, what matters here is not so much the actual number itself but rather how a worker *feels* that the wage she receives is good enough for her.

When chatting with a driver of a tour van in Iceland, I got a sense of calmness (not rushed, not resentful) toward foreign tourists like me, and of confidence in his government. During the drive, he told me how proud he was of how his government treated its new immigrants with care, providing them with good resources and opportunities. Once again, here, what matters is not so much whether or not the government actually provides new immigrants with good support but how the government makes the driver *feel* that it is taking care of these new immigrants that I find intriguing.

On a more random note, the same driver even gave me permission to use his music for my meditation audio for free—as it turned out, he is a musician. His assertion that he did not need money from me if I were to use his music was refreshing, considering that wherever else I went, everyone in the tourist industry seemed to always want a few extra dollars from us tourists. In other words, my encounters with workers in the tourism and restaurant industries in Iceland did not hinge on how much money they could get out of me. It was this pattern, in which they explicitly told me that they did not need money from me, that was different from most tourist places I visited. It made the power dynamic between the tourists and the workers more nuanced. This also made me wonder if there had been something that their government did to create such a public sentiment of contentment, and to manufacture a system of living that registered Iceland as the third happiest country in the world in 2017 (the year I visited), based on a report by the United Nations Sustainable Development Solutions Network.

My experiences traveling in New Zealand felt similar to my experiences in Iceland. It felt effortless, even as I traveled there alone and as a woman of color. Although they were not necessarily "warm and fuzzy" toward me, an Asian tourist in a country that had a history of being anti-Asian, people were accommodating and generally willing to help. When I wanted to do the Fiordland Jet, for instance, they were able to find a couple to go with me, so I was able to enjoy this thrilling experience. It might not be as profitable for them to take only three people on a ride (and I was the only passenger on the way back), but they were willing to figure out an arrangement that would work for me, as I told them that I really wanted to try their adventure but had to continue my road trip in the morning.

My week-long road trip in the South Island of New Zealand was wonderful. It began with a breakfast with my cousin and her two-year-old son at a place called Strawberry Fare in Christchurch. Their Ultimate Chocolate Dessert, which consisted of a brownie, chocolate mousse, chocolate ice cream, chocolate pâté, and raspberry coulis, indeed made for an ultimate breakfast. It gave a sweet boost to a morning that we spent mostly walking around town.

As the sun hunched over its midpoint, we walked back to my rental car. I gave my cousin one final hug, which felt as though I had just bitten a piece of extra dark chocolate with over 85 percent cacao, more bitter than sweet. I was grateful for the time lovingly spent, but did not know when we would see each other again—the joys and sorrows of being part of a big diasporic family, I suppose.

Inside the car, I held the steering wheel more tightly than I usually would. Anxious excitement filled me as I began the three-and-a-half-hour drive to Hokitika. I cranked up the music and with delirious ecstasy, offered my compliments—"Oh my God! You are SO GORGEOUS! I love you, I love you, I love youuuu!"—to the luscious-green and blue-sky beauty of New Zealand. The traffic was a breeze, as was the crisp wind that entered through my open windows. I hardly saw anyone on the road.

When I encountered people at the places I stayed or dined, I noticed that the people who worked there seemed to be chill and relaxed, not rushing each other, but not going the extra mile either. Perhaps because I mostly stayed in hostels and cheap motels, there was no extra friendliness that came with a price tag. But I always felt uncomfortable when the staff members at one of those expensive resorts greeted me with their pleasant and performative smiles anyway. The staff members at fancy hotels usually talked and moved with such trained elegance. Their meticulous eagerness to help was carefully cultivated to the point that it became seamless and natural. Sometimes, it even made me feel like I had just stepped inside the world of the *Stepford Wives* movie. As in the movie, this microarrangement and -management of the body of the workers functioned to signify their submission, in this case to the upper-class guests/tourists. Indeed, this is one of the ways in which class, power, and national hierarchies are maintained across national borders: through the disciplining of bodies.

The road trip itself was magnificent. From crossing the suspension bridge at Hokitika Gorge to hiking at Franz Josef Glacier to marveling at the beauty laid out so expansively underneath my feet at Lake Hāwea lookout, I felt deeply nourished. Going inside a dark limestone cave that was lit by bioluminescent glowworms at Te Anau made me feel as though I was back in Space Mountain at Disneyland, except the "attraction" here was one of nature, and it was not exactly a roller coaster as such. It was a soothing boat ride of being awestruck by the wonder of nature. Then, at Milford Sound, I went on a small cruise boat where I got to stand under the waterfalls and taste the glacial water. Needless to say, after a week of being enchanted by nature, I left New Zealand feeling lighter, as if my pain had reshaped its form into something fluffier and easier to carry with my body.

As I reflected on my visits to these countries, I came across a note in my journal that I wrote at the end of my trip to Iceland. It says, "There are two types of countries in this world: those where their people are rooting for each other; and those where people are left to fend for themselves and compete against each other." Surely, anything that begins with "there are two types of . . ." is always fraught with false oversimplification. Here, I invoke this personal note in my journal not to prove its truth but rather to get at the sentiment that I felt at that moment: I sensed that there was something larger, perhaps how a government ran its country and made its citizens *feel* taken care of, that might shape how citizens treated each other.

Certainly, I am aware that there are many layers that mediate the relationship between the government and its people, such as families, friends, the neighborhood we live in, the place where we work, etc. Yet, I wonder if national policies also influence how people treat each other and how they can relate to their family/children, workplace, etc., differently. For instance, I suspect that better paid-parental-leave policy at the national level would contribute to better relationships between parents and their children, as well as between parents-as-employees and their employers and other fellow workers, at the everyday level.

Let's be clear. I am not at all claiming that there is a causal relationship between New Zealand's and Iceland's national policies and my positive experiences in traveling to these two countries, where I observed people exhibiting a general sense of well-being and treating each other in a more supportive, rather than competitive, way. (I also am not saying that *everyone* in both countries I encountered was happy all the time.) Rather, my traveling to these two countries (and other places as a comparison) piqued my intellectual curiosity: What policies and programs do nation-states have when they prioritize their citizens' well-being?

The bottom line here is this: how people in Iceland and New Zealand treated me and how I, in turn, felt good and was better able to carry my pain when I was there, might be a mere coincidence. This experience led me to my story/theory but is not the story itself. My observation of how people acted toward each other in these two countries during my short visit was limited, and therefore could not be used as evidence for my argument. What my traveling to these countries and observing how people behave provoked me to do was to learn more about the policies and programs that focus on their citizens' well-being. After learning that there are, indeed, significant differences in the policies and programs related to the people's well-being in the countries where I felt people were more supportive of versus competitive with each other, I then theorized a concept that I call "emotional contract."

What the concept of emotional contract means at the nation-state level, why we need it, and what it may look like are the topics of this chapter. Of course, an emotional contract may look different in different countries. But the main message I want to get across is the same: if we want to carry pain in a more life-sustaining way, we need to have a good emotional contract with our government (or anyone in our lives, really). This is why we need to carefully choose where we live, as it influences how we carry pain in our lives.

Before I jump into the details of all that an emotional contract is about, I want to briefly reveal the subtext and context of when this chapter was written: during the early period of the pandemic in 2020. During that time, I read in various news outlets that Iceland and New Zealand were better able to crush COVID-19 in their countries. My experiences of traveling to New Zealand and Iceland help me understand why these countries, where the people I met seemed genuine in helping each other (and even me) and, most importantly, where the governments prioritize the well-being of their people rather than simply the economy, could come up with better and more holistic plans to handle the pandemic. In other words, although during my travels I had an inkling that there was something going on in these two countries that was different in comparison to the other countries I visited—this inkling made me come up with my "there are two types of countries in this world" note—I was not able to put it into words until after I read about how successful they were in handling the pandemic. Indeed, the pandemic shows how our lives could have been different if we had lived in a different city, state, or country.

I attribute Iceland's and New Zealand's success in addressing the pandemic to how they prioritize the well-being of their citizens. In fact, just a few months prior to the pandemic, in 2019, these two countries had announced these priorities. New Zealand's prime minister, Jacinda

Ardern, stated that New Zealand's politics would focus on "empathy, kindness, and well-being," and thus when a minister seeks approval for funding, they must prove that the suggested program will improve intergenerational well-being.[1] By the end of 2019, the prime minister of Iceland, Katrín Jakobsdóttir, joined forces with New Zealand's and Scotland's leaders to push for a "well-being" agenda.[2] It thus became clear to me that I needed to focus on these two countries as they would allow me to better illuminate and illustrate the concept of an emotional contract.

By October 16, 2020, Iceland had 3,929 cases and 11 deaths (32 deaths per one million population), and New Zealand had 1,880 cases and 25 deaths (5 deaths per one million population), compared to over 350,000 cases and 12,000 deaths in Indonesia (45 deaths per one million population),[3] and 8.2 million cases and over 223,000 deaths in the United States (674 deaths per one million population).

Moreover, because of how the United States handled the public health crisis, it was not a surprise that the *Washington Post* on May 26, 2020, reported that prior to the pandemic, about 25 percent of adults in the United States experienced "depressed mood"; this number increased to 50 percent during the pandemic.[4] The number was higher for women, poor people, and young adults, whereas those of high income seem to worry "half as often as the lowest" income group. This data shows, once again, that depression is shaped by class and gender status—it is structural, not just individual—and by the nation's inability to handle the pandemic in a way that shows that they care for their people's well-being. Thus, I want to emphasize that what matters is how the government makes its citizens *feel*, by way of the established programs and policies that show that they care about and are committed to their people. Emotional contract, operationalized through policies and programs, governs who gets to heal and who does not, and which bodies are left to die.

## The Emotional Contract and Gendered Politics of Emotions

I am offering the concept of emotional contract as a revision to existing social-contract theory. In a nutshell, what I want to get at is this: a social contract has been theorized within a masculine framework. Emotion, which has commonly been confined within the feminine space, is therefore rendered trivial in this masculine space, and overlooked in its articulation. To frame and demand an emotional contract from the government is to make visible and push for a revaluing of the gendered politics of emotion at a nation-state level.

Let's unpack this, layer by layer. A social contract, or the "original constitutional agreement," is a "fiction" that tells a story of the nation's relationship to its people and the terms of this relationship.[5] In this story, the nation enters into a relationship with its citizens in a "reciprocity of equals, each ceding to an equal degree his [*sic*] natural freedom to the state, and each receiving in turn its guarantee that his [*sic*] civil rights, liberties and property will be protected by its laws and decrees."[6] On the basis of this fictionalization, the nation justifies what is within the realm of its responsibilities to its people (e.g., to protect their property, etc.).

In this (original) version of the story, the social contract is problematic because only men are constructed to be citizens. That is, "only masculine beings are endowed with the attributes and capacities necessary to enter into contracts—only men are individuals. . . . The individual is constructed as a male body so that its identity is always masculine."[7] According to feminist political theorist Carole Pateman, because the social contract is imagined as a contract of equals only among men, another form of arrangement that she calls a "sexual contract" is made between women and men. This sexual contract governs "the legitimacy of men's power over women," which allows men to then enter into a contract with other men and the state.[8]

Not only is the social contract a contract of equals among men; it is also a contract of equals among white men. In *The Racial Contract*, philosopher Charles Mills points out that the social contract is not only gendered but also racialized, in that it "establishes a racial polity, a racial state, and a racial juridical system, where the status of whites and non-whites is clearly demarcated, whether by law or custom."[9] Nonwhite citizens are therefore not considered equal to their fellow white citizens, and thus are not entitled to the same protections as white citizens. Even when Jim Crow laws are no more and racial discrimination is indeed unlawful in the United States, the killings of Black bodies by police officers, as in the cases of George Floyd and Breonna Taylor, show us that the racist logic of the social contract is still operating even today.

When the social contract is understood as a masculine construction, care and emotion, which are constructed as feminine, remain outside of the social contract. This omission matters because well-being as something that citizens are entitled to and can demand from their government thus remains outside of the nation's domain and thereby its responsibility.

The logic goes like this: in a social contract, a citizen is constructed in masculine terms. The masculine concept of individuality is attached to the concept of "rationality," which is seen as the "enemy" of the emotional.[10] In the West, emotions are often considered as "irrational, uncontrollable, crazy, nonsensical, or useless phenomena" and therefore undesirable.[11] In this formation, "care and imagination" are undervalued, whereas "rational choice" is underscored.[12] Thus, if politics, citizens, and rationality are constructed as masculine, it is not a surprise that emotions and care, constructed as feminine, are left out of the articulation of nation, citizen, and politics.[13] The problem with this construction is that under this version of the social contract, men get a "pass" for not doing emotional and care work.[14] Women then have to bear the brunt of emotional work and "care activities inside and outside the market."[15]

This separation between politics and emotions, between the rational and the emotional, is what I aim to contest by highlighting the importance of an emotional contract.[16] The concept of an emotional contract recasts the nation-state as playing an important role in shaping its citizens' well-being and experiences of carrying their pain. It names and re-imagines the nation-state's relationship to its people as being registered at the affective level, and operationalized through national policies and programs that can affect people's well-being. Countries that consider the well-being of their citizens as a priority and recognize that the root cause of pain is oftentimes structural and political would have an emotional contract—by way of policies and programs that are put in place to help *democratize access* to well-being.

Emotion is political because it is part of a system that guides citizens to feel a certain way about an issue and as part of a nation/community.[17] To feel differently from the nation is therefore to be perceived "as a hostile threat."[18] For instance, if the nation's emotion toward immigrants is one that is negative, when some of its citizens embrace immigrants (think here also of immigrants with a particular race and/or religion deemed undesirable in this country), they will be perceived as a hostile threat to the nation. In this way, the nation does have the ability to impact its citizens' feelings and how they treat certain bodies and each other.

Given this ability, emotion can be registered as *an instrument of power* and an object of (national) politics. Ideologies are practiced and operationalized through emotions (i.e., ideologies regulate which emotions can be expressed, and to whom, who is allowed to express them, when, and in what context), among other mechanisms.[19] As anthropologist Bianca Williams sums it up so perfectly, "How we feel, how we understand our emotional selves, is influenced by politics and specifically systems of oppression."[20] Emotion therefore cannot be dismissed in the conversation about politics, the nation-state, and the social contract.

Thus, if I push for an emotional contract, I do so because it can provide us with the language to ask what protections from harm the state can be expected to provide its citizens. If the harm that women experience, such as from sexual abuse, is indeed structural, shouldn't the state be expected to protect its citizens from these harms? And, how can we hold the government accountable in their response to and responsibility for its citizens' pain?

To propose that well-being be framed as part of the social contract is to argue that well-being is systemic, structural, and political, rather than merely individual. To illustrate this point, it may be helpful to refer to feminist theorist Rosemarie Garland-Thomson's argument on disability as a "system of exclusions that stigmatizes human differences."[21] She argues that it is the system that considers certain body types as the norm/normal that creates specific technology that then *dis*ables particular bodies that are different from this norm. For instance, using a wheelchair itself is not a problem. It is only a problem when houses and buildings are constructed with stairs because they are built to only accommodate specific bodies that are deemed "normal," and disregard other bodies that are different from that norm. It is the stairs (the technology and the system) that *dis*ables the people; the people themselves are not inherently disabled outside this ableist system.

Similarly, in proposing the notion of an emotional contract, I am not concerned with what each individual affectively feels in their body, whether they are sad or happy, at a particular moment. People should be able to feel the entire range of emotions. What I am calling our attention to is how the system that is put in place makes it easier for certain people living in some countries to access well-being and *dis*ables others from accessing that well-being. These technologies and policies (e.g., the paid parental leave, healthcare access, etc., that I will detail below) can be a ramp that enables women, people of color, people with various mental health statuses, and poor, immigrant, and queer people to better access well-being. Or, the lack of these policies can function as the stairs that *dis*able marginalized people in their effort to achieve well-being.

Let this sink in: 75 percent of people in the world with a "mental disorder" do not receive treatment.[22] This shows that when a specific mental state is considered the "norm," the world is structured to exclude and stigmatize people who are psychologically diverse, rather than provide them with much-needed and accommodating access (through equitable policies and programs) so that we all can have equal access to well-being.

## The Emotional Contract Shapes National Policies and Programs

I begin with this premise: the country where we live matters to how we carry pain because the nation-state government *can*, if it wants to, guarantee *equitable access* to well-being for its citizens. Philosopher Jean-Jacques Rousseau stated that a social contract is useful for as long as it has "no other object than the general welfare" of its people. He wrote, "In order to establish a nation, it is necessary to add to these conditions one which cannot supply the place of any other, but without which they are all useless—it is that the people should enjoy abundance and peace."[23] That he explicitly stated the words "general welfare" and "peace" hints at the larger issue of well-being as something that should be included as part of the social contract. Remember, a social contract governs what a person loses and gains. When people enter into a social contract, they "consent to exchange their natural freedom for the order and protection a government supposedly can provide."[24] In other words, they lose their "natural liberty and an unlimited right to anything which tempts [them] and which [they are] able to attain," and in return, they gain protection of civil liberties and of property from the government.[25]

This "protection" that the government can provide in the form of programs and policies that focus on well-being is what I call an emotional contract. To give examples of what these programs and policies may look like, I turn to New Zealand and Iceland, particularly to the three areas that reflect the values of caring and care work (e.g., the paid parental leave policy); of being kind, generous, and empathetic toward stranger others (e.g., the new-immigrant programs); and of responding to citizens' perceived and potential pain (e.g., healthcare policy). By going through their policies and programs and providing just enough detail to show the differences among these countries, I hope to provide a better understanding of the emotional contract, so that we can demand that our government provide us with an emotional contract, too.

I want to clarify here that although I purposefully use the term "contract," I am not theorizing an emotional contract as an actual contract, bearing the weight of political and legal language. Rather, I frame it as a discursive or a "cultural rather than legalistic" concept.[26] This means that I do not use actual contractual language in this chapter. Nor do I propose an emotional contract to be a legally binding contract between the nation and its citizens—such a contract could manifest a different form of oppression wherein well-being becomes compulsory, and people who are not happy would be punished and ostracized. (It would make a good dystopian movie, though.)

I also want to make clear that in reflecting on these policies, I do not conduct a policy analysis or examine how they are implemented, as that is not my purpose. Rather, I offer this chapter as a theoretical think piece that allows me to revisit social contract theory, and consider these policies as a launchpad from which I theorize the notion of an emotional contract. Hence, this chapter may read more like a theoretical memo than an autoethnography.

## New Zealand

On May 30, 2019, Ardern launched the Wellbeing Budget, which allocates funding specifically to address issues of family violence, sexual violence, mental health, addiction, and the well-being of children and new mothers. With this budget, the state recognizes its responsibility for the well-being of its citizens and aims to address the issues that 27 percent of New Zealand children live in poverty and do not have access to healthy food, adequate healthcare, and a home,[27] and that 16 percent of the population has been diagnosed with depression.[28] In their efforts to boost mental healthcare, New Zealand allocated 1.9 billion NZD, half a billion of which goes to people who experience mild to moderate anxiety and depression but do not need hospitalization.[29] With this budget, New Zealand also hopes to integrate mental health workers in doctors' clinics, allowing patients to have a one-stop shop for mental and physical healthcare. The budget also funds a mental health support team at primary and intermediate schools, and "Sparklers," a program that allows educators to have access to online resources to help children manage stress.

## Healthcare

The New Zealand government provides healthcare access for its citizens, permanent residents, refugees, and foreign workers holding a visa for two years or more, which is publicly funded by taxes.[30] Under its national healthcare system, patients have access to free public hospitals—private hospitals and clinics are not covered. Primary care is free for children under thirteen years old.[31] There are copays that range from 15 NZD to 50 NZD, and for low-income people, the copay amount is capped at 17.5 NZD. Access to telephone health advice staffed by a registered nurse is free.[32] For prescription drugs, there is a 5 NZD copay for the first twenty drugs prescribed by doctors; they are free after that.[33] Dental costs are private pay, except for children up to eighteen years old, who may access free basic dental care through selected providers. Special services are provided to address health disparities among Māori and Pacific Islander populations, who have shorter life expectancies.[34] New Zealand also pledged 62 million NZD for mental health services provided to Kaupapa Māori and Pacific Islanders.[35] The program that targets specific populations is indeed necessary considering that based on 2017/2018 data, one in six adults experiences a mental disorder at some point in their lives, and marginalized people (women, Māori and Pacific Islander people, and economically disadvantaged people) experience more mental challenges than others.[36] Support services for disabled people are also available.[37] In addition to public healthcare, private health insurance is available, and about one-third of the population purchase it in order to have faster access to what is deemed nonurgent care.[38]

If I call Ardern's Wellbeing Budget a form of emotional contract, I do so because Ardern herself frames it as "a different approach for Government decision-making all together."[39] By way of an emotional contract, the government explicitly prioritizes the well-being of its citizens, and that is reflected in its allocation of funding. An emotional contract is the government's language of care. It speaks through policies and programs that allow citizens to feel that the government cares for their well-being, and provide citizens with structural conditions that make it easier for them to care for each other.

## Paid Parental Leave

Another policy that supports citizens' well-being is paid parental leave. In New Zealand, since the 1980s, women have had access to unpaid maternity leave. In 2004 paid parental leave became available.[40] Currently, parents whose baby was born on or after July 1, 2018, can get up to twenty-two weeks (continuously) of paid parental leave from the government; those with a baby born on or after July 1, 2020, can get up to twenty-six weeks. This leave is available for the parent (by birth, adoption, or "*whāngai*")[41] who will be the primary caregiver for the child until they turn six.[42] Under this program, an employee who has stopped working can get a maximum of 606.46 NZD per week before tax (in 2020), or a self-employed person can get either a minimum of 189 NZD per week before tax or up to 606.46 NZD per week before tax, whichever matches their weekly average earnings. Note here how the policy is straightforward, with clear definitions and parameters as to who can have access to this parental leave and what they will receive. (I will discuss more of the need for policies to be simple and straightforward in the next subsection.)

Also noteworthy here is how the campaign and debate that led to this successful expansion of paid parental leave from twenty-two to twenty-six weeks were framed through an understanding of the social contract. According to human development scholar Clare Mariskind, who examines people's online comments on the parental-leave debate in New Zealand, these comments range from citizens posting, "I do my best for this country, surely the country can do its best for my child" to "Most of these mums have worked their butts off, paid a lot in taxes over the years and deserve time off to raise their future tax payers" to "I don't see how anyone could turn this down, considering that we spend thousands to millions of dollars on roads."[43] These comments suggest an understanding of a social contract in which the government needs to be reciprocal in keeping its end of the bargain, after citizens have fulfilled theirs by paying taxes.[44]

### Programs for New Immigrants

In addition to caring for the new(born) members of its families by way of paid parental leave, New Zealand has also established programs to care for the new members of their country by way of new-immigrant programs. In welcoming their new immigrants, New Zealand funds the Citizens Advice Bureau (CAB) in thirty locations throughout the country, where new immigrants can speak to someone in person, often on a walk-in basis, to find out more information about living in New Zealand. The CAB also offers other services that help them settle in a new place, such as workshops, information sessions, and seminars for new immigrants.[45] I mention this without forgetting, however, that it was not until October 2019 that New Zealand ended a discriminatory and racist policy that restricted refugees specifically from Middle Eastern and African countries from moving to New Zealand.[46] We also should not forget Ardern's 2017 election campaign, which relied on cutting immigration by thirty thousand people per year.[47] In pointing out these seemingly contradictory policies (i.e., having a policy that would help immigrants settle in their new country, while simultaneously curbing immigration), I aim to illustrate how New Zealand strategically navigates and negotiates neoliberalism and the intermingling of race and immigration issues, as it reframes the social contract in emotional terms. To help make sense of this tension, and to avoid painting too rosy a picture of New Zealand, I invite the readers to read, among others, law lecturer Dylan Asafo's argument that the state has misappropriated and neoliberalized/individualized the "politics of kindness" to further marginalize Māori and

Muslim populations and evade the settler-colonial state's responsibility for its history of violence.[48]

## Iceland

### Healthcare

Iceland has public health insurance that is accessible to *all* legal residents who have lived there for at least six months, without any discrimination based on nationality. (Private insurance is available for those not covered by their public healthcare system.) Legal residents have access to free hospital and maternity clinics as long as the service is deemed medically necessary. The insurance also covers medically necessary visits provided by specialists, physiotherapy, X-ray exams, dental and orthodontic treatments for children and people over sixty-six years old, and "cash sickness benefits." There is a small fee for doctor visits, with clear schedules. For instance, a visit to the doctor during office hours is 700 kr (4.81 USD); a visit to an emergency room at a hospital is 6,868 kr (47 USD); and a laboratory test costs 2768 kr (19 USD). Monthly maximum out-of-pocket expenses are 26,753 kr (184 USD) per person, or 17,835 kr (122 USD) for pensioners, people with disabilities, and children.[49]

This seeming dream arrangement, however, does not cover visits to psychiatrists, as they are not part of the public healthcare system. People who cannot afford it therefore do not have access to psychiatrists.[50] There is a long waiting list for people to enter psychiatric wards.[51] The European Health Interview Survey of 2015 indeed reported that 9 percent of people in Iceland have "depressive symptoms."[52] Recently, however, there have been more "awareness programs" specifically promoting mental health programs run independently by groups such as Hugrún.[53] Certainly, an emotional contract must always include care for mental health treatments.

## Paid Parental Leave

Similar to New Zealand's, the Icelandic government also provides paid maternity/paternity leave and unpaid parental leave for its citizens. The maternity/paternity leave is given when a child is born, when a new adoption takes place, or when parents become new foster parents, for six months per parent, with six weeks transferable between the parents.[54] During this time, parents are eligible for payments up to 80 percent of the average income.[55] There is, of course, a limit to the minimum and maximum amount that parents will receive. In addition to maternity/ paternity leave, parents can take unpaid parental leave once, for up to thirteen consecutive weeks, before the child turns eight years old.[56] This policy indeed reflects how in December 2019, Prime Minister Katrín Jakobsdóttir explicitly stated that she prioritizes "green and family-friendly policies," instead of solely focusing on "economic growth."[57] Her focus on family and environmental well-being is another example of an emotional contract.

## Programs for New Immigrants

In terms of caring for new fellow citizens, the Icelandic government enacted an "explicit integration policy" in 2007. The program focuses "on democracy, human rights, social responsibility, and individual free-dom" for new immigrants. To this end, in 2009, the Association of Local Authorities in Iceland established a special immigration policy that "aims to protect immigrants' rights and teach them about their rights and obligations."[58] Legal-counseling and language-interpreter services are provided for free by the Icelandic Human Rights Office.[59] Also available are in-person programs such as Multicultural Centre/Fjöl-menningarsetur, which functions to facilitate "communications between individuals of different backgrounds, and to enhance the services pro-vided to foreign citizens residing in Iceland and to those interested in moving to Iceland";[60] Akureyri Intercultural Centre/Alþjóðastofa, which provides people with "information and advice regarding: education, social services, taxation, insurance, health services, courses in Icelandic, residence and employment permits";[61] and Women of Multicultural Ethnicity Network in Iceland, which provides peer support through its Women's Story Circle and other social events.[62] These programs function as elementary tools for new members of the nation, so they, too, can step into an environment where broader access to well-being is supported by the government.

## What Could Make It Even Better?

The above discussion on policies and programs in New Zealand and Iceland illustrates what governments provide their citizens with when they consider the well-being of their citizens to be a priority and recognize that the root cause of pain is oftentimes structural and political. Even then, the programs and policies that New Zealand and Iceland roll out in their countries only propel us to ponder more deeply about how to operationalize an emotional contract. They plot the possibilities of what having an emotional contract might look like. However, we need to push further and imagine what other spaces outside the dominant discourse can be incorporated under this contract.

For instance, rather than having national healthcare policy cover only "Western" medicine, we could initiate programs that include alternative treatments such as reflexology, massage, and acupuncture, etc., as well as healing foods and supplements, rather than only prescribed drugs. Instead of having new-immigrant programs that focus on simply integrating us into the capitalist and neoliberalist society as workers (e.g., in the form of helping us create resumes and find jobs), we should innovate programs that help immigrants feel that we are accepted in the new country, and that our belonging is not hinged upon our productive economic contributions to the nation (i.e., as good neoliberal citizens in a capitalistic system).[63] We need new-immigrant programs that would recognize and address how everyday racism can create an "ordinary trauma" in a diasporic family.[64]

## The Emotional Contract as Simple and Straightforward Policies

Policies and programs that are simple and straightforward are an essential part of an emotional contract. We need to remain skeptical of any nation that claims it prioritizes its citizens' well-being yet whose policies are not simple and straightforward.

To illustrate this point and provide a clear contrast, I turn to the two countries I have lived in and also visited during my sabbatical year (Indonesia and the United States) as points of comparison.

But first, I want to return to Iceland, for it was there where I realized that a sense of simplicity is crucial for our well-being. The first morning I was there, I went to a bakery for breakfast. As I was paying, I asked the cashier where the closest ATM machine was. She had to pause for a moment before asking her colleague, who then proceeded to tell me where it was. "I'm sorry, I forgot. We don't really use cash around here [in this country]. We just use cards for everything," the cashier explained herself.

"Really? No store has a 'cash-only' policy? So, I don't even have to go to the ATM, then!"

"Yeah. It's easy. Really simple."

Thinking back, I realize how simple and good an idea this is. It reduces the chance of the store (or people) being robbed; it also makes it easier for travelers not to have to find places to exchange or withdraw money. Of course, this also means making sure that all citizens have access to a (debit/credit) card as a form of payment, and that there is security in using the card. Thus, by "simple," I do not evoke simplicity in the false and nostalgic sense of "untouched by civilization," as one might fantasize about rural spaces in premodern times. Iceland is far from being "untouched" or "simple"—in fact, it takes quite sophisticated thinking to be able to streamline policies and modes of living in ways that contribute to people's well-being.

The idea that simplicity and clarity are essential for our well-being may seem obvious and commonsensical. Yet, prior to carefully going through the policies in these four countries (New Zealand, Iceland, Indonesia, and the United States), I was not aware of the extent to which the healthcare policies in Indonesia and the United States are convoluted and confusing, and may create the opposite of well-being: anxiety and frustration. For instance, I was frustrated when navigating the website of JKN-KIS (Jaminan Kesehatan National), the mandatory healthcare system in Indonesia, administered by the governmental body BPJS-Kesehatan (Badan Penyelenggara Jaminan Sosial), as it is not clear which information is located where. Even after I downloaded and read the entire 136 e-book pages that supposedly contain the important information, I still could not find all the data that I needed. This was in contrast to my experience of finding the information about New Zealand's healthcare on one succinct page online—it is succinct because the policy itself is simple and straightforward.

### Tiered System in Indonesia: Not Simple

In Indonesia, the national public healthcare system consists of three different classes of treatment, namely, first class, second class, and third class. The monthly premium that people have to pay depends on the class of treatment they want to receive. People who pay a first-class monthly premium, set at 160,000 Rp (11.45 USD), will receive first-class treatment at the hospital (with two to four patients in one hospital room);[65] the second-class monthly premium is 110,000 Rp (8 USD), with three to five people in one hospital room; and third class is 42,000 Rp (3 USD), with four to six people in one hospital room.[66] It is possible to upgrade to a better class, even if the person is paying a third-class monthly premium fee, by paying the difference.

These monthly premiums are only available for people who are not employees. Employees' monthly premium rate is calculated on the basis of 5 percent of their wage, with 4 percent paid by the employer and 1 percent by the employee. Veterans' monthly premium is 5 percent of 45 percent of their basic wage. For those who cannot pay the monthly premium, the government will step in and pay for them. Additionally, private insurance is available. Wealthy Indonesians at times opt to simply pay whatever price they have to pay in order to receive treatments by the doctor and hospital of their choice. Sometimes this means flying to Singapore, Malaysia, or Thailand to receive better treatments.

Unlike in Indonesia, public healthcare policies in Iceland and New Zealand are simple and straightforward as they do not have a tiered system wherein people with different jobs or economic backgrounds have different monthly premiums, choices, and medical treatments. In Iceland and New Zealand, people may have different copays, as detailed above, but the service is supposed to be equitable. *When the basic national healthcare system itself is already differential, it creates an environment where it is acceptable to treat people differently on the basis of their economic and class status.*

The problem with mental healthcare in Indonesia lies in the fact that not only does healthcare insurance not cover mental health treatments but also the number of providers itself is limited. According to WHO, Indonesia does not have enough psychiatrists: the ratio is 0.29 psychiatrist (in 2014) and 0.31 psychiatrist (in 2016) to one hundred thousand people.[67] According to 2018 data from the *Jakarta Post*, for Indonesia's 260 million population, there were only 773 psychiatrists.[68] Out of thirty-four provinces, eight do not have any mental hospitals, and three of these provinces do not have any psychiatrists; and out of forty-eight mental hospitals, half are spread out only among four provinces.[69] Part of the problem with mental illness in Indonesia is that people still believe that mental illness is a trivial matter that will go away on its own, or that it is related to the paranormal, ghosts, being cursed, or being punished, and thus instead of people with mental illness being taken to psychiatrists or therapists, they are taken to a *dukun* (shaman) to get rid of the curse.[70] This explains why only 9 percent of people who have depression seek treatment—there are 27.3 million people who have a mental illness, or about one in ten people.[71]

### Complicated System in the United States: Not Straightforward

In the United States, healthcare access is also complicated and convoluted. Under the Affordable Care Act (ACA) of 2010, health insurance became mandatory for all citizens and its costs are shared among the government, employers, and individuals.[72] Instead of being simple and straightforward, the seemingly expansive options for healthcare in the United States are actually limited and unaffordable/unequal. First, there is private health insurance, which is regulated at the state level. Then, there is public insurance, which consists of Medicare—a federal program for seniors over sixty-five and, to a certain extent, people with disabilities that is funded by payroll tax, individual premiums, and general federal tax revenues—and Medicaid and the Children's Health Insurance Program (CHIP) for people with low income, which is administered by the state and funded by federal and state taxes.[73] There is also the Veterans Health Administration and TRICARE for members of the military. Thus, except for Medicare, the United States does not have a national healthcare program. Most people (67 percent) have private health insurance, with the majority of them (55 percent) receiving health insurance through their workplace.[74] (Tying health insurance to one's occupation creates, rather than soothes, anxiety. It also makes access to well-being unequal.) This differential access to healthcare that is tied to employment and income inevitably creates a condition where people who have higher income live healthier and longer than those with lower income.[75]

On top of paying for monthly premiums for private health insurance, most patients have copays, with a set limit on certain out-of-pocket spending.[76] The rule for how much a person has to pay also differs depending on what service they receive, and where they receive it (in-network, out-of-network). I have private insurance, with 25 percent copay for most in-network services, through my employer. First of all, because my access to health insurance is tied to my workplace, I am limited in the kind of job I can choose. Secondly, with my current insurance, there are services that may cost me up to 40 percent in copays. My monthly premium for this insurance is about 150 USD a month. To increase my coverage so I could pay less, a 10 percent copay, I would have to pay almost 800 USD per month. This means that should something happen to me and I cannot pay my hospital bills, the government (as well as my family and friends) can easily blame me for not choosing a better insurance plan—the 10 percent copay—without considering that it is these choices themselves that are problematic and inequitable. Living in the United States makes me anxious about what will happen to me financially, if I ever fall seriously ill. Quite honestly, during the pandemic, I was more worried about the financial impacts of COVID-19, if I were to be hospitalized because of it, than its long-term health effects.

In the United States, there is a wide disparity of accessibility and quality of healthcare, especially among people with different racial and ethnic backgrounds, and certainly, income levels.[77] For instance, even when African Americans now have better socioeconomic status, they do not necessarily have better (access to) health.[78] Moreover, according to 2018 data, about 8.5 percent of Americans (27.5 million) did not have health insurance.[79]

For mental healthcare coverage, each health insurance plan has its own rules. Since ACA rules that mental health and substance abuse care are considered "essential," most health plans "cover preventive services and cannot deny coverage because of mental illness." Recently, there has been a move to integrate behavioral and primary care.[80] Nonetheless, the data shows that anxiety disorder is the most common mental illness in the United States, experienced by 19 percent of the population each year;[81] and about 31 percent of adults stated that they have experienced it at some point in their lives.[82] Out of those who have anxiety, only 36 percent receive treatment.[83] Of those adults who have depressive episodes, 66 percent receive treatment.[84]

This number is even bleaker when we enter gender into the picture. Women in the United States experience higher instances of anxiety disorder, about 23 percent, compared to 14 percent of men.[85] When it comes to generalized anxiety disorder, women are twice as likely as men to be affected by it. Women, more than men, suffer from posttraumatic stress disorder (PTSD).[86] The same is true of major depressive disorder (affecting about 8.4 percent of the adult population)—more women (10.5 percent) than men (6.2 percent) experience it.[87] These numbers show that mental well-being is gendered and systemic. Different expectations for women to fulfill their gender roles do create more mental restraint and issues for women.

### No Parental Leave: Leaving Parents Behind

In addition to failing to provide its citizens with a simple and straightforward healthcare system, the United States is the only country out of forty-one countries (including Estonia, Hungary, United Kingdom, etc.) that does not have any mandatory paid leave for new parents.[88] The other countries on the list give, at minimum, two months' paid leave. Indonesia is better than the United States in this regard, as employers are obligated to pay their female employees full salary for three months as part of their fully paid maternity leave (only 1.5 months can be taken after the birth; male employees are given only two days' paid paternity leave).[89] However, no policy is in place for self-employed parents or those who work for other people (i.e., domestic workers, etc.).

### No Programs for New Immigrants

There is no program in Indonesia for new immigrants. In the United States, there are a limited number of "free and low-cost" programs for immigrants, run by various nongovernmental organizations across the country that receive grants from USCIS.[90] As there is no standard for the kind and quality of services that these varied organizations offer—some are geared toward immigrants coming from specific countries, for instance—new immigrants do not have equitable access to these services and are left to their own devices.

## Conclusion: Where We Live Matters

Sociologist Tanya Golash-Boza asks this question: "Is simply being or becoming an American bad for your health?" Her answer: "It seems it might be, as the United States ranks fairly low for a country in the developed world on a wide range of health indicators. Moreover, immigrants often have better health than their native-born counterparts. In the United States, foreign-born women have substantially better pregnancy outcomes than women born in the United States."[91] This answer reflects how the United States, as the World Happiness Report documents, has become a "story of reduced happiness."[92] Indeed, its convoluted policies, which lack emphasis on the well-being of its citizens, as well as "declining social support and increased corruption,"[93] undoubtedly contribute to this story. Golash-Boza's answer is the verdict we all needed to hear loud and clear: where we live matters for our well-being.

To discuss pain without examining how the nation-state directly affects our capacity to respond to pain is to overlook one of the most important structures that determine our ability to appropriately address pain. Remember, the pain that we feel is also shaped by a larger system that structures our lives. At times, the nation-state not only fails to address the trauma of its people but is also creating more pain. For instance, data shows that almost 40 percent of people in the United States admitted to having politics as their stressor. Twelve percent claimed that politics affected their physical health negatively, and more than 4 percent of people reported feeling suicidal because of politics.[94]

This shift of focus from the personal/individual to the nation-state is meant to challenge the dominant and contemporary neoliberal view on how to deal with pain, which tells us that to change our lives, we need to change ourselves. By all means, we should feel free to keep improving ourselves. But as we do that, we need to also make sure that we have a supportive environment that makes individual changes possible and sustainable, and that access to healing and well-being are equal.

If this book makes the argument that we can carry pain in a more life-sustaining, humane, and feminist way, then, in this chapter, I shed light on the final question that we need to reflect on to do so: How does where we live matter to our pain? Here, I frame "where we live" within a nation-state context. However, I would encourage the readers to also evaluate the emotional contract that they have at all levels, from the closest circle, such as the people with whom they share the intimate space of their home (e.g., their life partner and family), to the neighborhood to the city to the state and to the country. In this way, we can use pain as an orienting tool that can tell us to move away from people and places that do not support us or make it possible for us to carry pain in a humane, life-sustaining, and feminist way.

## Theoretical Implications

For the readers who are curious as to why I propose the concept of emotional contract—what does this concept do?—I argue that the theoretical implication of reconfiguring the relationship between the nation-state and its citizens is to expand the meanings of citizenship. If Black feminist anthropologist and African diaspora studies scholar N. Fadeke Castor coins the term "spiritual citizenship" to name "the rights and responsibilities of belonging to community, informed by spiritual epistemologies,"[95] I propose the term "emotional contract" to flag citizenship as signifying not only national/political, cultural, or spiritual but also emotional relationships.[96] I redefine citizenship as citizens having a relationship, a contract, with their government that considers the importance of well-being. Considering citizenship as based on an "emotional contract" means that citizenship is an affective and embodied construction that is lived through daily practices and has consequences for how we live and carry pain in our lives.

Through the concept of emotional contract, I want to articulate a discursive narration of a nation that places emotion at the center of its social contract. In her book *Depression: A Public Feeling*, feminist theorist Ann Cvetkovich invites us to "think about depression as a cultural and social phenomenon rather than a medical disease."[97] I continue this trajectory of considering mental health as a social, cultural, and political issue by reframing well-being as something citizens attain as part of their social contract with the government. I contend that how a nation treats the pain of its people is revealing of its dominant political ideologies and cultural values: what and who it considers important and worth living a good, pain-free life. For instance, in a neoliberal and capitalistic country such as the United States, the government addresses mental health as a personal issue that needs to be dealt with at the individual level by way of therapy that individuals are responsible to pay for on their own. Oftentimes, the goal of therapy is to change the individual psyche without recognizing the need for ecological transformation.

Under neoliberalism, "personal responsibility" becomes a useful story because it lets the state off the hook. It allows the state to evade framing well-being as an object, a public good, so to speak, that the nation should also be responsible for. Demanding an emotional contract may pose a challenge for neoliberalism because neoliberal ideology creates self-invested and self-interested citizens who are unable to be cosufferers who can respond to the pain of others in a way that recognizes that pain is a result of systemic, social, political, and environmental toxicity, rather than simply bad personal choices or individual pathology.

An analogy might better clarify the concept of emotional contract. If psychology is a study that examines how parental/familial/childhood experiences contribute to one's psyche, a blueprint of human behavior, or well-being, an "emotional contract" is a concept that interrogates how the structural/the government (e.g., state policies and politics) contributes to one's psyche and well-being. This parallel between family and nation is not new. Some scholars have likened the "abandonment and denial of a country to its people" to "children's loss of a mother's protection."[98] Although such a parallel framing may be problematic as it once again normalizes the gendered heterosexual nuclear family that renders mother's love comparable to that of the now-feminized nation, what I am calling for, through the notion of an emotional contract, is a critical examination of the effects of a nation-state on its citizens' well-being. Through its policies and programs, the nation-state is providing its citizens with conditions of possibility within which to address pain. According to historian Julie Livingston, "Pain is a relationship . . . pain begs a response."[99] The concept of emotional contract invites us to think of a supportive and sustainable relationship between the government and its citizens, wherein citizens, considering that pain is the way of life, have the wherewithal to carry pain in ways that are more sustainable and humane.

My proposing that we need to demand that the government enter into an emotional contract with its citizens should not be registered as projecting my naiveté and idealism. Considering the current state of the United States, which is drenched with capitalism and neoliberalism, I am not at all optimistic that it will happen anytime soon (although it is currently carried out in New Zealand and Iceland, albeit in limited terms). My theorizing about emotional contract should not be read as my being a proponent of the nation-state as the ultimate form of governance either. I recognize that the formation and maintenance of the nation-state is often embedded in the history of violence.

Rather, by theorizing an emotional contract, I insist that we need to scrutinize the current social contract and renegotiate its terms to include our well-being. We must ask, Is the current social contract still acceptable for us when it is no longer "equal," not having the welfare of its citizens as its goal, and instead creates more pain in our lives? In this way, we need to recast the government as an entity that has the potential to be a coarchitect in building a structurally supportive environment where all citizens have access to a deeply satisfying life. If power can never be benign, can it at least ever be benevolent?

7

## Home(ostasis) Is Where the Heart Is . . . Healed

I end this book with a chapter that does not function as a concluding chapter for there can never be a conclusion when it comes to pain. There is never a finality to pain. Pain always finds a way to reemerge and undo what has been healed. I end instead with a meditation on home in order to offer a *sense* of completion. Almost every travel ends with a return home, even as future travels already lurk in the back of our minds, thereby mocking the very idea of a genuine completion.

In this final chapter, I share my thoughts in the form of multiple and disjointed vignettes, notes, and quotations to reflect the movements of thought and body during my year of travel. Although for some readers, this form of writing may feel jarring as it breaks away from the writing convention of the previous chapters, or even disorienting, as at times it feels like an unfinished (or lacking a clear) point, these snippets of thoughts and temporalities are what life, traveling, and theorizing feel like to me. This form also allows me to imitate my life's journey: life is not coherent. It does not have only one main point, one clear narrative, or one linear development. It may not even make sense. Life is scattered and experienced as small moments—hence the vignettes. Yet, every small point and moment is valuable, and contributes to the larger conversation this book is grappling with, on pain, travel, and feminist theory.

Part I. Home

*

If I were to choose an image that represents my life, it would be a labyrinth. It is but one twist and turn after another. Just when I thought I was almost there, so close to the center of the labyrinth, to my hopes and dreams, to healing, the path I was on took me further away from these things. But this did not make me give up hope. I have been walking in this labyrinth of life long enough to know that when I feel I am so far away from the center, the next turn might just suddenly take me right to where I wanted to be, if I just keep walking a little bit longer.

Sometimes I wish we could just take a shortcut and walk straight to the center of the labyrinth, without having to go through each and every one of its twisting paths. Is life not meant to be lived that way? Perhaps, we simply need to figure out what that shortcut is and how to take it.

All I know is that in this labyrinth of life, in its ultimate ending, we will return to the same place where we entered, our eternal home. One can only hope that it has been a truly fun walk after all.

*

After my year of travel was over, I came home to Hawai'i, a place that conjures up images of a picture-perfect paradise of blue sky, gorgeous turquoise ocean, and serene green foliage. The part of Hawai'i I came home to, though, was nothing of that paradisiacal sort. My small apartment was subsidized faculty housing, with old carpet and a toilet that backed up every three weeks or so. Ants marched neatly along my small kitchen windows. Roaches loved to play hide and seek in between the cracks of my kitchen cabinets. Right outside my window, exactly across from my apartment, the "Rainbow" campus shuttle made a stop every thirty minutes, picking up and dropping off students, staff, and faculty members, making tranquility and privacy a privilege and rarity. What was abundant was the unrelenting noise of screaming children and neighbors moaning from good sex. Lucky them.

*

Home was what I wanted to leave, what I left, and where I had to eventually return. For feminist theorist Sara Ahmed, home is a place one leaves in order to grasp the meanings of its existence.[1] Distance is supposed to give us a fresh perspective on home.[2] For Chicana feminist theorist Gloria Anzaldúa, home is something one leaves to "find [one]self."[3]

I did not leave home for the sake of knowledge, for I did not seek to know what home is or who I am. I simply wanted to be as far away as I could from (what I perceived to be) the site of wounding. Perhaps I thought that by traveling I could leave my pain at home for someone else to look after. But of course, we can never ask others to hold our pain for us. They do not know how to hold our pain in ways that will not hurt them, or us, even more.

But I wanted to leave home just the same.

*

November 2016, the night of the US election. A man who was anti-everything that I was—a queer/bi/wikisexual woman of color, an immigrant woman from the largest Muslim country in the world—was projected to be the winner. I sat at the beach with a blank gloomy stare. The orange-red sun was about to set over the shimmering blue ocean.

It was then that I knew that if my sabbatical request was approved, I would travel the world for the entire year. I wanted to be anywhere but here, where my world was burning raspy fire at its center.

*

To return is thus to resent home. *Is it not?*

*

The Unpacking.

A black convertible dress that can be worn in twenty different ways (e.g., as a dress, a skirt, a top, a pair of pants, etc.).

A couple of sweatpants and t-shirts that can function as an exercise outfit, sleepwear, or casual wear.

A raincoat.

A swimsuit.

A nice dress.

A work dress.

A silk travel liner.

A snorkel and a mask.

A few sets of underwear.

A pair of walking sandals.

Travel-size toiletries.

Travel documents.

Basic makeup kit.

A pair of flats.

A smartphone.

An adapter.

A nice top.

A laptop.

I emptied all these items from my carry-on bag. A carry-on bag and a handbag were all I carried during my travels. That is how I usually traveled, for a year or a weekend. Light, indeed. It was cost efficient, too, since each checked suitcase would add thirty-five dollars or more to each leg of the trip.

For everything else heavy or bulky, like a jacket, a sweater, a scarf, a long-sleeve shirt, a hat, or a pair of tennis shoes, I would simply wear them.

My small suitcase was my sidekick, the one to stare me in the eye and tell me not to buy every beautiful trinket I saw while traveling, *No space, no more space!*

My sidekick made unpacking a breeze.

*

The Unpacking: The Saga Continues.

New friendships.

New memories.

New routines.

New me (?).

New pain.

New hope.

New dream.

What else?

The gems of intangible items;

the kind of souvenirs that won't fit into a box.

I wonder: How does one unpack them?

I wonder, too: Are tangible items easier to unpack because they can be contained in a suitcase and therefore seem manageable, and are visible and therefore categorizable (i.e., I can return them *to* where they physically belong, with other items in a similar category)? Are intangible items therefore harder to unpack because they are infinite and invisible (i.e., functioning as my ghostly sidekick), and because, whether or not I am aware of their presence, they are returning home *with* me, altering the very landscape of my behavior, identity, and home?

A return *to* versus a return *with*.

A return *with* signifies the need to make space for and sense out of them, the intangible items, my ghostly sidekick.

A case in point: I wanted a new routine that I learned during travel to be a part of my life at home. So I *tried* to go to the farmers' market more often, to replicate those experiences I had in Kotor and Madrid. In the beginning, my shopping basket was brimming with mangoes, oranges, and starfruits. When I was feeling a bit more ambitious, I would even add choy sum, celeries, and cucumbers into the mix. But without the sweet smell of ripe fruits to greet me, not to mention the inconvenience of driving to the farmers' market, I stopped going regularly. I failed to make space for this new habit I had picked up during travel. Yet, it did not feel right to just give it up. (And so the saga continues . . .)

My ghostly sidekick made unpacking a beast.

*

To return home after traveling the world without changing anything about the home is to continue to carry pain in the same way. One must heal the home, if one wants to heal at all.

Home matters in our relating to pain because it is in the home (however it is defined) where we first learn how to carry pain in a certain way.

*

The meanings of home have been defined and redefined in paradoxical and contradictory ways. Home can be understood as "both nostalgia and resentment"; "belonging and alienation"; "both a haven and . . . a site of oppression"; both "strange and familiar"; simultaneously "stable," "fixed," and "bounded" and "flexible," "messy, blurred, and fluid"; both "spiritual, healing, and transformative" and "a site of disappointment, betrayal, violence, anguish, and uncertainty"; "both comfort and conflict, as well as raced, classed and gendered"; and both safety, "security and comfort" and a space of trauma, especially for women.[4]

Home also stands for "a narrative history, . . . a social identity," "social bonds," "memory," "idea and hope," "anticipation and promise," "feeling(s), practices," "a safe, often feminine sphere," "that place which enables and promotes varied and everchanging perspectives, a place where one discovers new ways of seeing reality, frontiers of difference," and a "physical geography."[5] Home can work "as theater and as play, of place and of process or experience"; it can be "multiple, fluid, transient, provisional, a process; a verb."[6] One can even be "an exile" "from oneself at home."[7] Home can be "unhomely."[8]

So many meanings, so little understanding.

But when Driftpile Cree Nation writer Billy-Ray Belcourt likens the "reserve" to a "morgue" and to "body bags" and "call[s] it home anyways,"[9] I cannot but ask, *For whom do the meanings of home matter? For whom is home impossible?*

*

Home can be an identifier of a place where you are from or where you live, but it should never be your identity.

*

Home does not even have to "be conceived of in territorial terms at all."[10] It can also be registered through its "temporal contingencies."[11] Scholars Mitra Etemaddar, Tara Duncan, and Hazel Tucker coined the concept "moments of home," which "points to the period of time where one or more of a combination of different and fluid components of home can cause diaspora to feel as though they are 'at home.'"[12] These components of home can range from "the presence of close family, friends, or a certain category of people"—which Etemaddar and colleagues emphasize as more important than "the place of that [family] reunification"—to "familiar habits and smells" and to being "anchored in certain objects."[13]

When my brother and his wife came to visit me to celebrate my birthday in Budapest, home was indeed built on old stories, familial feelings, and familiar objects.

*

Home can also be a healing space.[14] In some hospital discharge instructions, home is even listed as "the ideal site of return."[15] Feminist theorist bell hooks writes, "We can make homeplace that space where we return for renewal and self-recovery, where we can heal our wounds and become whole."[16] Some homes can indeed be healing. (But some other homes may need healing.)

*

If home is really where the heart is . . . healed, and where the self is consolidated,[17] then, I may never be healed . . .

(Some people are forever searching for their "home.")

*

In the beginning of my travels, I had a deep longing for home. One of my secret (and perhaps silly) goals, to travel to as many countries as I could during my sabbatical year, was to find a country where I could eventually retire—to find my "forever home." I have lived in three countries: Indonesia, Canada, and the United States. I feel at home in none of them.

*

The first country I visited during my year of travel was Indonesia. It was the place not only where I was born and raised but also where the annual writing retreat for women in academia that I cofacilitated took place that year. At the end of my retreat, my cofacilitator and I stayed a few extra days there, in Bali.

That night, I had my nice dress and makeup on. I was thrilled to take my cofacilitator/dear friend to a fancy restaurant in town, showing off that this "third-world country" has a fine-dining restaurant that is more over-the-top than those in the United States.

I arrived at the restaurant with an empty stomach, but full of excitement and high expectations.

"The dining area is full, but you can still have dinner at the bar," the host told me with a smile, as she elegantly deflated my excitement. I told her I would ask my friend first before deciding if we still wanted to have dinner there. *Why didn't I make a reservation?* I blamed myself.

My friend was waiting at the bar while sipping a lovely-looking drink. "Sure," she calmly replied. She was always easy-going like that.

"Is that the friend you're going to have dinner with?" the host asked me after I told her that we wouldn't mind having dinner at the bar.

"Yes . . . , yes, she is," I answered hesitantly and walked back to the bar.

A few minutes later, the host approached us and told us that as it turned out, they had a table in the dining area available for us after all: for me and my white friend.

Unwelcomed in one's own home, except when dining with a white friend.

Yes, I knew that home could be a site of wounding, "of racism, sexism, and other damaging social practices."[18] Yet, it was still a hard pill to swallow when it happened.

I was no longer in the mood to show off. Trying to boast that racism in Indonesia is better or worse than in the United States is not that appetizing a subject.

*

The second country I visited was France. Renzo, my partner, joined me there to watch the spectacular Fourteenth of July fireworks, which were indeed magnificent. As we were leaving the country for our next destination, Prague, we were waiting at the check-in line at Paris Orly airport. A person watching the line waved his hand, alerting me to go to the available check-in desk. I was walking toward the only desk that was open. Renzo barely moved. He was walking rather slowly behind me, creating a big gap between us.

The woman behind the check-in desk signaled me to go somewhere else.

"Where?" I asked, as I got closer to her.

"Over there."

I walked away to where she was pointing, although I couldn't see any available agent. "But there's nothing else that's open," I told her from where I was standing.

She shrugged her shoulder, "You're not my client. He's my client."

She pointed to and waved at Renzo to approach her. He then began walking toward her. I stood there in the middle of no one's line, all confused. As she was talking to Renzo, who now stood right in front of her counter, I walked back to where they were.

"Oh, you're together?" She looked at me doubtfully, then forced a smile rather awkwardly. "I'm sorry . . . I didn't know."

No longer at home in Indonesia, but not being served by another woman of color until I have a white companion, just the same. The color blindness of racism. You can be a racist no matter what your skin color is.

Is this what Anzaldúa means when she writes, "Wherever I go I carry 'home' on my back"?[19]

*

For an immigrant, one's "features, appearance, and accent" become one's home.[20] Our body is our ultimate home: "No matter what passport one carries, the body that looks 'foreign' is subject to a variety of gazes—from the curious and rude to the dangerous and violent."[21]

*

Home reveals the limits of humanity and the violence of ideology.

To long to own a home is to dream the capitalist dream, to be under the capitalist magic spell. For as long as we own a home, we cannot say that we live a life that reflects our againstness of capitalism, of borders. Home is the very manifestation of a border, between oneself and one's neighbors, enabled and fueled by capitalism. We shall never forget that "homely-homes are utopian, bourgeois, idealized, and indeed Eurocentric."[22]

*

Yet, I dreamed of owning my very own home, just the same.

Each time I visited a new city during my travels, I updated the list of things I wanted for my dream home. At first, I wanted a home with a million-dollar view, like that from the London Eye, but without the million-dollar price tag. I wanted to be enchanted by the view every single day. I also wanted a home in a vibrant city where I could walk to cute cafés, fresh and flaky croissants, and magnificent museums, as in Paris. But then, I went trekking in the Himalayas, and added "proximity to the healing miracle of nature" on my list. The ultimate dream, of course, is to have a home in a country that has an emotional contract with its citizens.

Good luck in finding such a place, especially on my professor in women's studies' salary.

*

Home is but a story I keep revising in my head.

*

A homestead in the head—in memory and the imaginary, is always accessible. The question is, Which device do we use to take us there?

During my year of travel, ramen noodles were a sure tool to take me "home." No matter where I was, as soon as I found a good ramen noodle place, I would feel less restless and more grounded/at home. When I was in Fukuoka, Japan, I was staying at a nice hotel for a workshop, but the food in the surrounding area was not much to my liking. Whenever I had a free afternoon, I would go to the 7-Eleven in the city, the only place I knew that sold Michelin star Nissin instant tantan ramen in a cup, and buy nine packs of them. I would eat it every day. (The health-conscious reader might cringe here, and I understand their feeling.)

When I was in Madrid for the first time in October 2017, I would go to the same ramen restaurant, Ramen Kagura, and wait in their long line to get the same kind of tantan ramen noodles. (When I came back in the spring, they told me tantan ramen was only served in the fall, so I stopped going.) In Calgary, I would go to my favorite ramen restaurant, Tsikiji, and get its tantan ramen. In Sydney, it was Ryo's noodles in Bondi that would transport me home.

That Japanese ramen noodles were my way home, although I did not grow up in Japan and never stayed there long enough to affectively register Japan as my home, speaks to the rootlessness and multiplicities of home.[23] As some scholars point out, home exists in "multiple locations" and can be registered as "a plural notion."[24] It was in Indonesia, where I was born, that I first learned to love Indonesian instant ramen noodles

(*SuperMi*). But it was in Hawai'i, where I currently live, that I became addicted to Japanese ramen noodles. This means that for me, the feelings and "moments" of home can be accessed anywhere in the world, as long as I can get my hands on a bowl of slurpy good ramen noodles.

*

But home can also be a cruel invention. For it seeks to tell me that I do not belong. Here. There. Anywhere.

If home is too cruel, too contradictory, too settler-colonizer-y, then, healing cannot be about going/finding/having (a) home.[25]

## Part II. Home(ostasis)

* *

Healing is "the broader restoring to wholeness (whether or not a 'cure' is effected as well)"—whereas being cured is "the elimination of a disease as defined by the biomedical system."[26] Psychological healing is similarly understood as "a process of . . . restoration of or return to the patient's true or real self [. . . to] restore psychic wholeness."[27]

To prime the conditions of possibility for "self-healing" is to return to homeostasis.[28]

* *

Homeostasis is "any self-regulating process by which biological systems tend to maintain stability while adjusting to conditions that are optimal for survival."[29] Home is only optimal for healing when it functions as or can create homeostasis.

* *

*Homeostasis, not home, is when/where healing happens.*

* *

When I am at my homeostasis, I begin to carry pain differently (see chapter 5).

I begin to understand how pain can feel so personal, although it never was.

"Why me?" is never the question.

Sometimes we want to know the why of pain so we can do the how of healing.

*But there is no why in pain.*

All of the stories. None of the answers.

* *

Homeostasis is not (about pursuing) happiness.

Happiness hoists you. Sadness sinks you. Homeostasis is emotions melting into each other and unto themselves.

Happiness cannot be the goal of healing, of life's journey, because "the face of happiness" often "looks rather like the face of privilege."[30]

* *

When I am at my homeostasis, I can feel it—the "quietness of joy." I feel alive. Yet, I feel calm at the same time. The paradox of homeostasis bliss.

* *

I found my homeostasis in Vienna, Austria, where life was about coffee and cake. The kind of sweet life I dreamed of. Mornings were spent waiting in line to get a table at my favorite coffeehouse, Café Central, and writing a book, while sipping Viennese-style iced coffee with whipped cream, and layering my ideas with a slice of the cake of the day.

Afternoons were spent walking around town, visiting museums, from the Belvedere Palace, where I was enchanted by the original *Kiss* by Gustav Klimt, to Sigmund Freud's museum, where I wondered why some homes could make their occupants such daring thinkers.

Nighttime was filled with music. Sometimes, the Mozart concert at the Golden Hall; other times, the brilliant jazz performance at Club Porgy and Bess.

In Vienna, I was animating, intimating, and mending the spirit. I came into embodiment with that which enchanted my mind, body, spirit.

My homeostasis.

* *

Healing—homeostasis—is conversing with one's own mind, body, and spirit. It is poking around at the edges of knowing, of feeling. I have yet to find a way to shorten the conversation.

I cannot remember when I started this conversation with my mind/body/spirit. I only remember that it has involved psychotherapy, psychiatry, biofeedback therapy, shamanic healing, reiki healing, Vipassana meditation, Theravada meditation, Osho meditation, guided meditation, yoga, Pilates, belly dancing, zumba, acupuncture, cupping, reflexology, Hawaiian spiritual healing, lomi-lomi massage, deep tissue massage, network care, chiropractic, fascianator/rolling, juice diet, vegetarian diet, and many different forms of food supplements (from spirulina to organic B12 to organic cat's claw to vitamin micro-C to vitamin D to organic nettle to ginseng to curcumin to MSM to lysine to magnesium glycinate to organic cranberry to barley grass to organic zinc to lemon balm to ashwaganda to red marine algae to red clover to aloe vera juice to licorice root). Judging from this long list, you can tell that I am (perhaps over?) committed (or addicted?) to healing and finding my homeostasis.

To converse with and listen to my body required that I try one new healing modality or take one new food supplement at a time, and see how my body responded before committing to it. Trying one thing at a time as a form of listening to my body perhaps started with the biofeedback training therapy that I was doing when I was living in Kansas. My therapist attached electrodes to my skin to monitor my blood pressure and my heart and breathing rate. He would try one different healing modality each week, and see whether or not that particular method improved my vitals and emotions. He also gave me a small tool, called a "stress thermometer," to practice biofeedback therapy at home. (These days, smart watches, such as Vivosmart 4, have a function that tracks our stress level all day.)

I vividly remember watching an episode of *Grey's Anatomy* while being hooked up to my stress thermometer, and being surprised to see that my stress level went up. Seeing my body respond to a television show, something that was not even real, was the evidence I needed to believe that it did not matter whether or not the trigger was real, or whether it related to my life; the affective effect was similar. I have since been more careful about curating which news or social media postings I engage with, as they may bring unnecessary stress into my life and disturb my homeostasis. This means that I also have to curate my friends list, online and offline, because healing requires that we have a good "social support (i.e., being cared for)" system.[31]

* *

Because healing involves having a good support system (think here of emotional contract—chapter 6), it is not solely about taking on personal responsibility to keep "working" on ourselves.

During my sabbatical year, I went on a few cruises: along the Mosselle River (from Strasbourg to Trier), the Amazon in Peru, and the Galápagos Islands in Ecuador. These were relatively small cruises, with sixteen to fifty passengers. All three companies did a good job of making me feel at home, although in my own home I did not have anyone cooking me meals or doing a turn-down service and leaving chocolates on my nightstand or a towel in the shape of a monkey on my bed. That surely made life on a cruise easy and enjoyable. Going on a cruise made me realize that healing (and even living) is about *showing up, enjoying the show, and going with the flow.*

Yet, our neoliberal- and capitalist-infused friends, families, and societies teach us that to heal, we need to do the work, mostly on ourselves, no less. When the concept of homeostasis is translated through neoliberal language, it is articulated through the rhetoric of having a work-life balance, pursuing which will create more anxiety and pressure than homeostasis.

Being on a cruise awakens me from this neoliberalistic dream: healing *requires* nondoing and, in some cases, unlearning. It is about returning to wholeness—homeostasis. To heal is to stop trying too hard and stop trying to please others. Pleasing others is not the same as serving others. Serving others comes from a space of having a full, filled, and fulfilled heart. Giving from the overflow. Pleasing others comes from an empty space of wanting others' hearts and loves to fulfill my own. My ultimate pain-making machine.

* *

The question is thus not *where is home?* but *what is my homeostasis?*— "my" because to each their own. One's healing potion can be another's poison.

My daily regimen of healing potion is having sixteen ounces of organic celery juice every morning on an empty stomach. This practice, popularized by Anthony Williams, the author of the *Medical Medium* book series, has been criticized for not having scientific backing and causing some side effects for certain people. (It certainly troubles the boundaries between what counts and does not count as "medicine.")

The great thing about training myself to listen to my own body instead of other people (with or without scientific backing) is that if it sounds intriguing and safe, I will try it for myself, at least for thirty days. For me, this daily practice of celery juicing works. After a year of consistent celery juicing at home, my blood tests for cholesterol, diabetes, kidney, and thyroid came back normal. My anxiety level also became more manageable on most days. (All I need to do is to continue this practice diligently, which I must admit has not always been easy.)

* *

If home is "a way of life, a way of being, a culture, a way of thinking,"[32] then *homeostasis is a way of being, thinking, and living that is optimum to one's life.*

If "home" is a word we use to convey a level of intimacy with someone—for which room in our home we let someone into exposes the level of intimacy we have with that person (e.g., the bedroom versus the living room, etc.)—then homeostasis is about having the right person enter the right room.

Homeostasis is aligned intimacy.

* *

Home turns into homeostasis when it is built on *habitable places and healthy habitual practices.* Turning a place into a home involves "home-making" and "place-making" processes, which incorporate "embodied practices that shape identities and enable resistances."[33] People are incorrectly labeled as "homeless" (or, the correct term, "unhoused") because their home is considered uninhabitable and deemed unhealthy by society.

* *

Some places make it easier for me to create healthy habitual practices and reach homeostasis than others do.

During my travels, I noticed that where I was staying shaped how I acted and behaved—my habits (see chapter 5). I suppose this is why we have to carefully choose where we live: a place has the power to turn us into a different person—even the kind that we might not like. Feminist researcher Saba Gul Khattak writes, "Leaving home is thus not a simple act of changing one's place of residence. It denotes a parting of ways with a life that one is familiar and comfortable with."[34]

When I was in Jakarta, I became a different person. I was lazy—having domestic helpers who would do everything for you, from your laundry to driving you places, could do that to you. I noticed that my friend, a sweet and stylish woman I met randomly on a train in the

Netherlands almost two decades ago, also became a different person. She was criticizing and raising her voice to the receptionists at her doctor's office in Jakarta. "If you don't yell at them, they don't listen to you," was what she told me when she noticed the surprised look on my face. There, my days were filled with going to shopping malls, dining out, and meeting one friend after another who talked about expensive handbags or cars. Class status mattered a lot. Perhaps when you live in a country with poverty as the norm, acting rich makes you stand out.

In Sydney, where I stayed with my uncle, I had different habits. I would wake up early in the morning, around five, and meditate for at least fifteen minutes in the company of the Buddha, and the gods and goddesses of Rama, Sita, Sri, and Saraswati. I would write for two hours and then jog around the neighborhood, making a stop at the free gym in the park. Some late afternoons, I would walk to the river and sit on one of the benches until the sun hid behind the high-rise apartments. I love watching sunsets. It reminds me that the sun will set on its own time. It cannot be rushed, and it won't wait for anyone else to show up before performing its mundane miracle.

Once a week, I would go with my uncle to Eastwood market to buy fresh strawberries, watermelon, grapes, oranges, peaches, or kiwis. I would look up websites that listed local events and go to see some shows and art installations. I didn't do any of this in Jakarta. I felt more at my homeostasis in Sydney than in Jakarta.

* *

*The hard and simple truth is: homeostasis is possible wherever we are.*

Traveling helps make visible what needs to be shed to return us to homeostasis, but it is an unnecessary and expensive device. Other devices discussed in this book, from shifting our perception (chapter 3) to working with our body (chapter 4) and to practicing feminist enchantment in our daily lives (chapter 5), are accessible tools that can be employed anywhere, anytime.

True, traveling may be beneficial when we need some time to un-plug, from work, our mundane daily routines, or people we love but who overwhelm us. But there is no place in the world that can be far enough for us to forget our pain or fix our problems. We carry them with us everywhere we go.

* *

And there is another use of traveling.

Traveling transnationally may allow us to expand our limited catalog of emotions and find new ways to feel and new feelings to experience. Sociologist Xavier Escandell and anthropologist Maria Tapias point out, "As migrants encounter new opportunities or hardship, or negotiate new power relations, they are exposed to new emotional vocabularies and ways of 'feeling.' The longer they stay abroad, the more acquainted they become with 'new' ways of expressing emotions and the more they have to reconcile these views with the emotional knowledge they carry. At times this reconciliation entails adopting new modes of expression and may cause more distress as migrants 'second guess' their original beliefs about emotions; at others, they may remain steadfast in their original beliefs."[35] Although this book does not explore migrant experience, it nonetheless attempts to show how traveling to twenty countries in one year led me to find "new emotional vocabularies and ways of 'feeling,'" particularly, of pain (see chapters 3–6).

* *

Traveling also helps me meditate more deeply on pain.

I ask, Whose scars, whose wounds, whose pain am I really carrying? What new methods of carrying pain can I employ? How can I cultivate more generosity toward pain, toward myself, toward the stories I do not know yet how to tell about my pain? Have I learned to treat pain with the softness, gentleness, and kindness that it deserves?

I see: . . . (like the three dots that appear on my phone as the other person is typing, and I await the answer with much anticipation and anxiety).

## Part III. Returning Home, Returning to Pain

\* \* \*

The final editing of this book takes place as Russia has just invaded Ukraine, and Western Australia has reopened its border for international travels (which had previously been closed due to the pandemic). Together, these two events foretell an increased movement of bodies across national borders: some will be forced to flee their beloved homes, and some others will return home to be reunited with their families. And there are others still who will fly to follow the paths of exquisite and enchanting images on Instagram (I surely have been guilty of this myself).

At this time, the pandemic has been raging for more than two years, and thrown me into a world of disenchantment (where my practice of feminist enchantment was abruptly disrupted). It has jolted me into a way of existing in which I am not quite sure how to inhabit both this new world and my body—a feeling of not being at home in my body, and simultaneously of not being in my body while being at home. It creates in me a barren longing to be with other bodies, to escape the boredom of being bound at home, and to marvel at the beauty of foreign and faraway landscapes.

It also makes me wonder what the future of travels will be like. I worry that the pandemic will widen the gap between those who can pay for COVID tests, international health insurance, extra days to quarantine at a government-approved hotel, increased prices of almost everything, and those who cannot. I writhe in agony over the pain we feel at the hands of the various levels of government with whom we have no emotional contract, as they dole out new restrictions for how to travel, how to embody our bodies, and how to live our lives.

What, then, can we make of this pandemic-magnified pain?

\* \* \*

Pain as a transnational feminist object, an anamorphic apparatus, an orienting tool.

Beyond these fancy concepts, I contend that pain remains *a way for the body to pitch its stories to us. What we do with these stories determines how we carry pain in our lives.*

We need to take note of what pain tenaciously tells us to move away from. As an orienting force in my life, pain has indeed taken me far, to twenty countries in one year, and to different embodied feminist practices. Pain has pushed me away from the people, places, and habits that wound me. I know of no other phenomenon that can demonstrate tough love better than pain.

\* \* \*

As an anamorphic apparatus that I carry during my travel, pain has allowed me to see and theorize differently about perception (chapter 3), embodiment (chapter 4), enchantment (chapter 5), the social contract (chapter 6), and homing/healing (chapter 7).

\* \* \*

When it is not suppressed, repressed, or denied, pain has the potential and power to deliver on its premise and promise: that pain is here to alert and orient us, to launch us into emotional, physiological, spiritual, and intellectual adventures toward our homeostasis haven. Pain is an irrefutable force to be reckoned with in our lives and in our theorizing feminism.

Indeed, this book is offered as a call to embrace the elegance and eloquence of pain, as an attempt to ask more about and from pain (e.g., by positioning pain as a transnational feminist object), and as an experiment with what to do and how to do things with pain (e.g., by my employing transnational feminist autoethnography).

By posing the key questions that guide our journey with pain, this book also serves as an invitation for others to conduct their own "experiment" in how to experience, think about, and live with (or carry) pain differently, each time it shows up in their lives. It is my hope that this book can push us to make more audacious demands of our pain and ask bigger questions about pain: What *can* we ask from pain? How can we be more creative and courageous in carrying pain in our lives?

* * *

I have breathed through different kinds of pain. Some of which, I have graciously exhaled. Much more of which, I will surely inhale, but not just yet. What I dread is no longer the pain itself but the empty spaces and the gentle pauses in between pain that may be filled with fear, worry, and sorrow—mostly, my own, but also, others': What will my pain do to others, their feelings, their well-being?

In the end, there will be pain so great we will no longer know how to carry it. Even our body will yield to it, passing up the opportunity to figure out a better way to carry it, passing it away. But that time has yet to arrive. In the meantime, just as author Anne Lamott teaches us that writing happens "bird by bird," so we need to always remember that living, too, happens pain by pain. And in some odd ways, that is truly the gift of life.

# ACKNOWLEDGMENTS

This book was conceptualized during many moments of listening to Krista Tippett's *On Being* podcast, and being intrigued by her question of how we can live differently. In this book, I engage with her question and translate it as, "How can we live with pain differently?" I am grateful for and inspired by her deep, thoughtful, and thought-provoking work.

Claire Moses has been, as always, the first person to hear about and read the entire draft of my book. She embraced my plan to mix various genres and encouraged me to stay true to that desire. Without her fierce brilliance, tireless guidance, and overflowing generosity, this book would simply not have been written in the way that it is. I thank her profusely, and with so much love.

The reviewers of this book have been generous and meticulous in sharing their extremely thorough and helpful feedback. They truly are dream reviewers—I could not have asked for better reviewers! Thank you to my editor at NYU Press, Ilene Kalish, for finding these reviewers. She has been supportive and enthusiastic about my project from the very beginning. It truly has been amazing to work with her. The *entire* team at NYU Press has always made publishing such a fun and superproductive endeavor. I thank them all enormously and expansively, to the moon and back.

These beautiful and brilliant souls have read various parts of my book and provided me with spot-on, much-needed, and gratefully received feedback: Chandra Decker, Heather Rellihan, Tanya Golash-Boza, Neha Vora, Joanne Rondilla, Christina Lux, Anna Stirr, and Lissa Manganaro. Vernadette Gonzalez has also patiently listened and suggested some thought-provoking ideas whenever I vented about the difficulty of writing this mixed-genre book. Her genre-busting books have been influential in my life. I am deeply grateful for her encouragement and brilliance. I am also indebted to my editors, Wendy Bolton and Meghan Drury, who have handled this book with so much care and meticulousness.

My truly supportive colleagues at the University of Hawai'i at Mānoa, and my Indonesian communities in Honolulu and beyond, make my (academic) life less isolating and more delicious. I am grateful for each and every one of their friendships.

Sibling love is the kind of love that sustains me from the inside. And this is only the case because I get to have Agung Nugrahaeni and Ibnu Magda as my siblings. These two incredibly talented young women have also given me hope for the future: Annette Archaeni and Diza Edgina have been my portals to anything smart, cool, and hip. I love and thank them oh so, so much, as much as my heart can handle.

To the readers and my communities of practice: Thank you for creating a safe space for my book to land. May the healing journey be beautiful and kind to us all.

An earlier version of chapter 4, "How Can I Work with My Body to Process Pain?," appeared as "Why Non-Story Matters: A Feminist Autoethnography of Embodied Meditation Technique in Processing Emotional Pain," *Women's Studies International Forum* 73 (2019): 1–7, and is reprinted with permission from Elsevier. The seed of this article was written during a writing fellowship at Faber Residency in Olot, Catalonia. I am beyond grateful for the generous support.

# NOTES

## CHAPTER 1. ALL ABOUT PAIN

1 Certainly, these are not the only questions we should be thinking about. As others travel and discover more questions for all of us to consider, I would be eager to learn about and meditate on them as well.

2 Michelle Leve defines neoliberalism as "a political-economic ideology and practice that promotes individualism, consumerism, deregulation, and transferring state power and responsibility to the individual" (Leve, "Reproductive," 279). In this book, neoliberalism is an important concept because as American studies scholar Catherine Rottenberg argues in her book *The Rise of Neoliberal Feminism*, neoliberal ideology produces the imperative to be happy. Happiness is seen as one's personal responsibility, attaining which requires the individual to invest in themselves by way of self-care activities, for instance. This means that even healing one's pain becomes one's sole personal responsibility.

3 Of course, if the readers have the means to travel, even just to the next town or province, I would always encourage them to explore the spaces beyond their comfort zone and embrace the unknown. I am not at all saying that people do not need to travel. I am saying that people can still shift their relationship with pain, even when they cannot travel due to physical, financial, emotional, legal, or other restrictions in their lives.

4 Cohen et al., "Reconsidering," 2. Also note that the word "pain" has its root in the English word "*poena*," meaning punishment (Wall, "On Pain," 58). In ancient time, pain was believed to be a punishment, a bodily invasion by "evil spirits"; to avoid it, a person must be faithful and seek protection from the Divine Spirit (Cohen et al., "Reconsidering," 5). "Pain" is often coupled with (or juxtaposed to) the word "suffering," whose root word is "*sub-tire* (bearing)" (Wall, "On Pain," 58). Although pain is often seen as more objective, while suffering is seen as more subjective, such a distinction may not be useful in understanding pain in philosophical terms (Wall, "On Pain," 58). Pain is also differentiated from trauma: "While pain is often traumatic, trauma is not necessarily physically painful" (Murray, "A Postcolonial," 7).

5 Wall, "On Pain," 58. Indeed, in its modern conceptualization, pain is understood not as a "thing" or "disease" in itself but rather as "an experience" (Cohen et al., "Reconsidering," 2, 5). Pain has also been seen as a bodily occurrence, an affective state existing at the "presymbolic, or imaginary, level where the hierarchical

organization of language still has not taken place" (Olalquiaga, "Pain Practices," 263).

6  Ahmed, "Contingency," 18.

7  Valentine, "'The Calculus,'" 30.

8  Bost, "Gloria Anzaldúa's," 22. For the definition of "affect," I follow Teresa Brennan, who defines it as the "physiological shift accompanying a judgement" (Brennan, *Transmission*, 5).

9  Anzaldúa, *Borderlands/La Frontera*, 27. Similarly, critical legal theorist Illan rua Wall points out that to understand pain as the way of life is to grasp how pain "*is* the very hard wiring of our bodies, . . . There is no 'pain centre,' there is no place in which the 'objective' pain ends and the 'subjective' suffering begins" (61). He also emphasizes that pain is "the fundamental trait of the soul's nature. Everything that is alive, is painful" (Wall, "On Pain," 60). Life without pain is thus nonexistent.

10  Bost, "Gloria Anzaldúa's," 26.

11  Bost, "Gloria Anzaldúa's," 25.

12  Anzaldúa, *Interviews/Entrevistas*, 276.

13  Contemporary feminism has also revolved around "the expression of pain, the pain of a female body in patriarchal culture" (Forte, "Focus," 252).

14  hooks, *Yearning*, 215.

15  Pain is also what feminism makes visible. Feminism alerts us to what is wounding at the site of transnational hetero/patriarchy. Pain's relationship to feminism, however, is not always productive. For political theorist Wendy Brown, demanding political rights by insisting on evidence of suffering of the self is concerning as the sufferer becomes "invested in its own subjection" (Brown, *States*, 159). Here, pain becomes a "'wounded attachment' that inadvertently preserves rather than challenges the point of injury" (Philipose, "The Politics," 64). Moreover, in feminism, pain in the body often becomes a site to construct a victim subjectivity (Orlan, "Intervention," 318). This victim stance is criticized for at times painting a picture of the victim as "pure innocent" and the perpetrator as "pure evil" and suggesting that "suffering can be ennobling" (Gilmore, "Agency," 89; Murray, "A Post-Colonial," 4).

Other scholars, however, even while taking Brown's warning to heart, have offered different and, I believe, more nuanced approaches to pain and subjectivity. International politics scholar Liz Philipose, for example, points out the difference between "embodied pain" ("subjectivity is constituted in pain or . . . the self is constructed through emotion") and "victimization" (Philipose, "The Politics," 64). She argues that articulating an identity that is based on pain does not necessarily mean taking a victimized stance, because the act of articulating that very pain is already an exercise of asserting one's agency and making meaning of pain (Philipose, "The Politics," 64). Artist Bill Burns, communications researcher

Cathy Busby, and communications studies scholar Kim Sawchuk similarly argue that "asserting that one is in pain is not a declaration of victimhood or self-pity, or 'the new narcissism,' but an acknowledgment that we are not independent agents in absolute control. We inhabit pain-filled environments" (Burns et al., *When Pain*, xxii). In this approach, articulation of pain does not necessarily indicate a subjectivity that is attached to being wounded. I agree with theorist bell hooks when she argues that we need to avoid a feminist identity that is based on shared victimhood, or a feminist subjectivity that arises out of being in pain (*Feminist Theory*). We must not, and need not, fetishize the wound or forge an identity that relies on being wounded to demand social justice. To read more on this, see Saraswati, *Pain Generation*.

16 As such, I expand the previous understanding of pain as "a linguistic object" that provides us with "a way of being and a way of speaking about the world" (Miles, *Pain*, 1). Moreover, feminist theorist Sara Ahmed leads the way in shifting the question from what pain is to what pain *does* (Ahmed, "Contingency," 22). In this way, we can understand pain as an instrument, although not necessarily in German classicist aesthetics' sense of a means to "obtain harmony and wholeness" (Lyon, "'You,'" 31). It is this notion of pain as an instrument, particularly as a theoretical and transnational feminist object, that I explore in this book.

17 Women's studies scholar Leigh Gilmore, drawing from philosopher Bruno Latour's network theory, develops an understanding of (chronic) pain that appears as "an actant sharing a body with another actant who has memories and consciousness of a life before pain, who is suffering, and who seeks to end pain. . . . If we call pain an actant, it is not to foster conditions in which it thrives. Rather, it is to note the ways in which pain places a demand upon a person and impels her toward accommodations, re-orients life and life narrative, and exerts a lively presence" (Gilmore, "Agency," 92).

18 The author would like to thank Diza Edgina for this metaphor.

19 Ahmed, *The Cultural Politics*, 27.

20 Zaner, *The Context*, 54. Moreover, pain, functioning as *of* the body, but not *in* the body, creates a "double alienation" (Leder, "The Experiential," 453). As "interior to the self," pain is "unshareable" and "inexpressible," making the sufferer feel alienated from oneself, in addition to from others; as "threateningly exterior," pain "has the power to disintegrate our customary sense of relationship to others and our own embodiment" (Leder, "The Experiential," 453–54).

21 Scarry, *The Body*, 52.

22 One of the values of pain throughout the history of Western medicine is that it functions as "a symptom of an underlying injury and disturbed bodily function," and carries with it "a threatening reality" (Cohen et al., "Reconsidering," 4).

23 Svenaeus, "The Phenomenology," 111.

24 Goodeve, "You Sober People," 230.

25  Latino/a studies scholar Suzanne Bost argues, "Pain signals a threat to the system, a challenge to that which we perceive as 'normal' corporeal states" (Bost, "Gloria Anzaldúa's," 22).

26  Brabant, "Reflections."

27  Quoted in Fitzpatrick, "What She," 87.

28  Williams, *The Pursuit*, 11.

29  In academia, travel writing as an insightful genre for knowledge production began to gain currency after Edward Said's *Orientalism* was first published in 1978. Travel writing functions as an important site of knowledge production as it "generates a complex system of cultural representation" (Kaplan, "Hillary," 5).

30  Dubrov, "Rational," 98.

31  Dubrov, "Rational," 98.

32  Dubrov, "Rational," 95. This anamorphic apparatus "combines different strands of scientific rationality in order to allow an image of the sublime to appear. The image itself is very real, but it is, in effect, empty if we cannot understand that it is the result of many different apparatuses of culture, language and technology" (Dubrov, "Rational," 96).

33  New Scientist, "Anamorphic Art."

34  New Scientist, "Anamorphic Art."

35  Of course, pain can help us understand many, many other crucial things in life—whatever "X" we fancy, so to speak. I focus on these main questions as they have overlapping practical and theoretical significances for my book.

36  Here, I am echoing anthropologist Bianca Williams, who argues, "Feeling, emotion, and affect are forms of knowledge. They provide ways of knowing the world and figuring out how to navigate it" (Williams, "The Pursuit," 37). Similarly, sociologist Ghassan Moussawi points out, "Bad feelings orient us toward new questions, objects, and subjects of analysis" (Moussawi, "Bad Feelings," 93).

37  Hood, "Re-Articulating," 6. In the field of pain studies, feminist philosopher Elaine Scarry's *Body in Pain: The Making and Unmaking of the World* has been foundational in framing pain as something that "contracts and negates," lacks creative powers, is "world-destroying," and is "an expression of negation and annihilation," which she juxtaposes to "imagination [that] is expansive and explores alternative realities" (Scarry, *The Body*, 29, 168–69; Bost, "Gloria Anzaldua's," 26). Indeed, the traditional view of pain within human rights discourse is that pain is seen as something that needs to be solved and avoided (Wall, "On Pain," 67). Moreover, most scholarly studies on pain have been framed through discourses of disease (Newmahr, "Power," 389).

The exception to these works that frame pain as negative are literatures that focus on voluntary pain, that is, in extreme sports or in sadomasochistic (SM) practices (Newmahr, "Power," 391). I take note here of the words of cultural historian Celeste Olalquiaga, who argues that in SM practices, pain is turned into "a positive experience of individual development and is often lived within a group and in a ritualistic context" (Olalquiaga, "Pain Practices," 263). In this context, pain is celebrated as a distinct experience that can only be surpassed by an even more painful experience (Olalquiaga, "Pain Practices," 263). Cultural anthropologist Margot Weiss, analyzing SM communities in the United States, focuses on how pain becomes the circuit of the commodity exchange in these communities (Weiss, *Techniques*). Yet, even the scholarship that shows how people embrace pain still acknowledges that pain is mostly viewed as negative. For example, in her ethnographic study of SM communities in the northeastern United States, ethnographer Staci Newmahr finds that although some SM practitioners see pain as more positive—they like to feel the hurt, a category of pain that she calls "autotelic pain"—they still see pain as carrying some negative weight, which she distinguishes into three different categories: "transformed pain" (pain is unpleasant but it can be transformed into pleasure), "sacrificial pain" (pain is undesirable but it is necessary for a greater good), and "investment pain" (there is a payoff in experiencing pain) (Newmahr, "Power," 389–411). Hence, she concludes that pain is still "*understood and experienced as inherently and originally negative*" (Newmahr, "Power," 389, emphasis in the original).

38  Stanford, *Bodies*, 15.

39  In refusing to dichotomize psychological and physical pain, I want to make clear that I do not lump all pain together. The origins, intensities, and symptoms of pain may indeed differ from one person to the next, from one moment to another. I do not mean to imply that pain can mean anything and everything so that it becomes meaningless, a signifier without signified. My reframing of pain as a transnational feminist object is meant to point us to a new direction for how we understand pain, and how we can live with it differently. I recognize that for some people, my book about my experiences of pain may not resonate with the pain that they are currently feeling.

40  Goodeve, "You Sober," 230.

41  Bost, "Gloria Anzaldua's," 27.

42  By connecting the body to its environment, I want to evade a possible misreading of feminist enchantment as solely a personal or, worse, a neoliberal practice.

43  By bringing in and emphasizing emotions in the conversation about the social contract, I thus revisit and revise existing scholarship on social contract theory.

44  A note of genre clarification: I hope it is clear that this book is not and should not in any way be categorized as "travel writing" per se, or, at least, not in its traditional sense. Travel writing often has as its goal "the production of difference; we read travel writing to read about an other place or people" (Ramos, "Literary," 150). This book's alignment with the travel writing genre is in the fact that this book *inevitably* produces knowledge about the places and people that I encountered during my travels. This book remains wedded to proposing new theories about pain as its main goal, however.

CHAPTER 2. ON THE METHOD OF TRANSNATIONAL FEMINIST
AUTOETHNOGRAPHY

1 This effort has increasingly been more solidified by the affect theory turn in the humanities.

2 See Clough, "Autotelecommunication," 101.

3 I develop this method by building on the pioneering works of feminist autoethnographers and paying a transnational feminist attention to pain. In this book, I frame the body-in-pain as a gendered body, and assert that what creates the pain to begin with is often structured by an ideology of gender as it intersects with other articulations of power (e.g., race, nationality, etc.)—and power that flows transnationally.

4 Naber, "How to Name."

5 Saadawi, My Travels, 27.

6 Naraindasa and Bastos, "Introduction," 1.

7 Winet, "Toward," 34, 167.

8 Theorists Cherríe Moraga and Gloria Anzaldúa coined the term "the theory in the flesh" and defined this theory as "one where the physical realities of our lives—our skin color, the land or concrete we grew up on, our sexual longings—all fuse to create a politic born out of necessity. Here we attempt to bridge the contradictions of our experience. . . . We do this bridging by naming our selves and by telling our stories in our own words" (Moraga and Anzaldúa, "Entering," 23). I also appreciate author Nikki Lane's definition of the flesh as "living, breathing, and acting bodies" and as referring "simultaneously to issues of embodiment and the way bodies are engaged in theory and practice" (Lane, "Bringing," 647–48). Transnational feminist autoethnography values an embodied approach. It takes seriously the materiality of the body and bodily experiences and aims to produce "sensual theories," where "mind and body emerge from one another" (Chawla and Rodriguez, Liminal, 1). This means that transnational feminist autoethnography is mindful of how "power operates through affect" (Grossberg quoted in Harding and Pribram, "Losing," 872). To follow the flow of power is to trace the movement of affect and emotion.

9 Travel can indeed be used as a distraction from "the pains and trials of one's situation" (Bardwell-Jones, "Travel," 5) and a way to "escape spatially and temporally from anxieties, pain and dislocation" (Alù, "Fabricating," 290).

10 As John Lyon argues, "Meaning does not inhere in pain, and so both observer and sufferer must impose meaning onto pain. Moreover, pain and its visible referent, the wound, demand interpretation. . . . We want it to mean something, yet for it to mean anything, it must belong to a narrative, and so we create narratives to attribute meaning to pain, to make our bodies signify" ("'You Can Kill,'" 33).

11 Mukherjee, The Emperor. This shift in the behavior of the cells can be likened to how "the 'ecology of the self' is restructured with a change in the environment" (Stefan Hormuth quoted in Roberson, Defining, xvii).

12 Kelleher, "This Is Your Brain."

13 Lambert, "The Bloom Effect."

14 Crane, "For a More Creative Brain."

15 Franklin and Crang, "The Trouble," 7.

16 The word "travel" is related to the French word "*traveiller*," which means to work or "to labor" (K. Siegel, "Women's," 57). Indeed, prior to the Enlightenment, travel was seen as an arduous journey that a person had to endure, and was associated with "suffering" or "a penance" (Leed, *The Mind*, 5; K. Siegel, "Women's," 57). Traveling as suffering was often employed as a narrative device to emphasize and frame the importance of the hero in the story (Leed, *The Mind*, 6). In this sense, travel functions as a "test" of one's character, revealing who the person truly is when they have nothing else but themselves, and have to endure trials and tribulations during their travels (Leed, *The Mind*, 6). During this time, especially the fourth to fifteenth centuries, the most common traveling figures in Europe were "the scholar, the crusader, and the pilgrim" (Smith, *Moving Lives*, 1). During and after the Enlightenment, travel took on new and multiple meanings. For instance, as transnational feminist scholar Inderpal Grewal points out, during the eighteenth century, young men of the aristocratic class began to take the Grand Tour for educational purposes (Grewal, *Home*, 1).

   Travel also has many, many other meanings. They range from "colonizing" to "a means of social and ideological transformation" (Schweizer, "Political," 19) to "a pleasure and a means to pleasure" to "a means of discovery, of acquiring access to something new, original, and even unexpected" (Leed, *The Mind*, 5) to a process of "self-discovery through a search for an absolute other" (Birkeland, *Making*, 33) to "a process [of] creating individuation and autonomy, and identity formation" (Birkeland, *Making*, 64) to a "practice of re-centering oneself and casting off anxieties attached to one's identity" (Dubrov, "Rational," 13) to an "individual choice [that] is considered to be an activity one does alone to achieve self-transformation" (Bardwell-Jones, "Travel," 23) to a "way of thinking about the transitory nature of mobile identities in a transnational world" (Bardwell-Jones, "Travel," 163) to a way of attaining "new experience" (Saadawi, *My Travels*, 214) to "escaping the self" (Dubrov, "Rational," 14) to providing the momentary abandonment of "one's ideological conditioning" and increasing one's ideological awareness (Schweizer, "Political," 103, 118) to a form of "translation" (Euben, *Journeys*, 43) to "find[ing], creat[ing] and remak[ing] western selves" (Birkeland, *Making*, 33) to "a means to discover enchanted aspects of the modern world and of the self" (Dubrov, "Rational," 14) to "an act of learning how to perceive objects, and an object that alters perception" (Dubrov, "Rational," 12) to "a praxical activity that deeply informs the ways in which we are social" (Bardwell-Jones, "Travel," 9) to "an act that spurs writing" (Dubrov, "Rational," 15) and to "*theôria*" (Euben, *Journeys*, 28).

17 Pitugshatwong, "Crossing Boundaries," 3.

18 Alacovska, "Genre," 133.

19 S. Mills, *Discourses*, 27.

20 Pitugshatwong, "Crossing Boundaries," 14.

21 Pitugshatwong, "Crossing Boundaries," 15.

22 Pitugshatwong, "Crossing Boundaries," 3.

23 Smith, *Moving Lives*, xi. More specifically, modernity here refers to "democratiza-
tion, literacy, education, increasing wealth, urbanization and industrialization,
and the colonial and imperial expansion that produced wealth and the investment
in 'progress'" (Smith, *Moving Lives*, xi).

24 Pitugshatwong, "Crossing Boundaries," 3. Travel writings during the colonial
period (including those written by women) were important as they functioned as
"an instrument within colonial expansion and served to reinforce colonial rule
once in place" (S. Mills, *Discourses*, 2).

25 S. Mills, *Discourses*, 121; Alacovska, "Genre," 133. In highlighting the gendered
aspect of travel and travel writing, I think it is important to note here that in the
epic story of Gilgamesh, travel functions as "the medium of traditional male
immortalities" (Eric Leed quoted in S. Smith, *Moving Lives*, ix). "Good travel" is
"'heroic, educational, scientific, adventurous, and ennobling'" and "'is something
men (should) do' while women travel only 'as companions' or 'as exceptions'"
(Clifford, *Routes*, 31; Alacovska, "Genre," 133). When it comes to travel, "men were
the spiritus movens of the public sphere and were destined to 'mobility'—to act,
to progress and to move" (Alacovska, "Genre," 133). Travel is even seen as
"constitutive of masculinity, and it is the very antithesis of femininity. By
implication, the genre of travel writing becomes 'an androcentric' genre—a genre
of male identification that disqualifies women from participation and even
pathologizes femininity" (Alacovska, "Genre," 133). Travel writing thus "embodies
the 'masculine' pretensions to rigour, 'objectivity' and 'truth'" and "has been the
preserve of the well-heeled, muscular and educated man" (Alacovska, "Genre,"
133). In the 1930s, travel was used as one of the ways in which a man proved his
manhood (particularly for English authors) (Schweizer, "Political," 76).

26 S. Mills, *Discourses*, 35. These writings also function as a way to "disciplin[e]
non-Western territories" (De Mul, *Colonial*, 22).

27 Catherine Stevenson quoted in Smith, *Moving Lives*, xi.

28 K. Siegel, "Women's," 57. The tourist figure is often criticized for operating from
the perspective of a "Eurocentric gaze" and embodying the "agonistic traveler"
(Holland and Huggan, *Tourists*, viii; Lugones, *Pilgrimages/Peregrinajes*, 82). The
Eurocentric gaze "perpetuates colonialism—even imperialism" and has "ethno-
centrically superior attitudes to 'other' cultures, people, and places" (Holland and
Huggan, *Tourists*, viii). The agonistic traveler, according to Lugones, is "a
conqueror, an imperialist. . . . Their traveling is always a trying that is tied to
conquest, domination, reduction of what they meet to their own sense of order,
and erasure of the other 'world'" (Lugones, *Pilgrimages/Peregrinajes*, 82). The

tourist figure is often problematic as it functions as a way to measure one's self-progress/transformation against the other (Winet, "Toward," 18). Yet, the figure of the tourist allows us to better understand meanings of "citizenship," "consumerism," "cosmopolitanism," "globalization," and how "transnational modern life is organized" (Winet, "Toward," 30).

29  Butler, "Global Chicks," 2.

30  Butler, "Global Chicks," 2–4, 28. The global chick figure embodies "empower-ment" and "choice" and "may articulate critiques of orientalism, imperialism, and/or the suffering wrought by economic globalization. Most importantly, she is distinctly not a tourist, and not a colonial adventurer" (Butler, "Global Chicks," 3).

31  Saraswati and Shaw, *Feminist*, xv. To employ a transnational feminist analysis is thus to "focus on movements across borders (that of people, ideas, time, and feminism(s)) as well as avoid the traps of feminist orientalism, or the idea that Western feminists can travel around the world applying their own perspectives to other peoples and cultures (a kind of travel enacting one's own imperialism in the name of personal or gender liberation)" (Winet, "Toward," 52).

32  Grewal and Kaplan, "Global Identities," 48; Tambe, "Indian Americans," 468.

33  Saraswati, *Pain Generation.*

34  I want to evoke here the brilliance of Intan Paramaditha in her article "On the Complicated Questions around Writing about Travel," in pointing out how Indonesians or third-world subjects have become foils for white feminists to articulate their agency.

35  For instance, these white bodies get to be "expats" while we are called "immi-grants." And whereas our bodies are considered as nondesirable in these spaces—or only desirable under certain predicaments of work, sex-work, etc.—the presence of white bodies may increase the rent value in a neighborhood deemed worthy for "expat living," etc. I am pointing this out to make visible the class aspect of racial categories.

36  Grewal, *Home*, 3.

37  Kaplan, *Questions*, 23.

38  Kaplan, "Hillary," 236.

39  Alexander, *Pedagogies*, 4. To address this issue, Lugones suggests that as travelers, we do not perceive other people/cultures with an "arrogant eye," that we become aware of the systems and privileges that allow us to travel to different "worlds," and that we stay away from wanting to search for that which is "authentic"— which she suggests is "a self-regarding, narcissistic search from a position of power" (Lugones, *Pilgrimages/Peregrinajes*, 28). (Note that the "world" here does not necessarily mean different countries, but rather, the differential spaces of power.) When we travel, it is also important that we employ a "feminist travel gaze," which is defined as "inversion of the gaze in travel," "embodiment of race and other physical markers," "awareness of gender and constructs of gender, masculinity, and sexual preference," "understanding of networks of power,"

"recognition of the construction of nationalism," and "unwillingness to accept 'a single story'" (Winet, "Toward," 96–97).

40  Bardwell-Jones, "Travel," 6; Williams, "The Pursuit," 9.

41  To learn more about wikisexuality, read Saraswati, "Wikisexuality."

42  I want to pause here for a moment to complicate how I use the word "privilege." I want to divorce privilege from its dominant meanings of "unearned." Often, people provide a narrative that works to counter their white privilege by saying, "I work hard. It doesn't come easily for me." Whether "unearned" or "earned," privilege can still be problematic. Thus, I use the word "privilege" to mark my relational and intersectional locations of power and access to resources, be they earned or unearned.

43  K. Bhattacharya, "Autohistoria-teoría," 198.

44  Ellis et al., "Autoethnography," 1. More than simply a method, autoethnography can become

> a way of being in the world, one that requires living consciously, emotionally, and reflexively. It asks that we not only examine our lives but also consider how and why we think, act, and feel as we do. Autoethnography requires that we observe ourselves observing, that we interrogate what we think and believe, and that we challenge our own assumptions, asking over and over if we have penetrated as many layers of our own defenses, fears, and insecurities as our project requires. It asks that we rethink and revise our lives, making conscious decisions about who and how we want to be. (Ellis, "Preface," 10)

45  Bochner, "Putting," 53; Chawla and Atay, "Introduction: Decolonizing," 4.

46  Stewart, "An Autoethnography," 659.

47  Adams et al., *Autoethnography*, 1–2. Also see Toyosaki and Pensoneau-Conway, "Autoethnography," 561–73.

48  Bacon, "Narrative," 132–33; Jackson, *Paths*, 4.

49  Laura, "Intimate," 289. As English literature scholar Zoë Kinsley argues, it is about valuing "the role of the individual traveler as the perceiver and verifier of external data" (Kinsley, "Narrating," 74–75). Moreover, in recognizing the situatedness of the traveler, autoethnography also affords me an opportunity to illustrate why certain ways of processing pain may work for me but not for other people, and the micro ways in which pain works.

50  Vidal-Ortiz, "On Being," 181.

51  Vidal-Ortiz, "On Being," 199.

52  Clough, "Autotelecommunication," 174, 179.

53  In weaving travel and theory production, I am intrigued here by the ancient Greek practice of *theôria*, which refers to how "the acquisition of knowledge requires not detachment from the world but movement in and through it" (Euben, *Journeys*, 28). *Theôria* connects "travel, direct experience, and vision" (Euben, *Journeys*, 27). Although the Greek practice of *theôria* is "the etymological

precursor to the English word theory," the terms "*theôria*" and "theory" should not be collapsed or conflated with each other (Euben, *Journeys*, 27–28). Historically, "*theôria*" was used in its early days in Herodotus's *Histories* and is "tied specifically to the achievement of knowledge" (Euben, *Journeys*, 27). At the time, "carefully selected" travelers ("men of good repute over the age of fifty") would travel for a maximum of ten years and when they returned, they had to "be rigorously examined" and "the knowledge they br[ought] home carefully vetted by those presumably capable of distinguishing between wisdom and contamination" (Euben, *Journeys*, 27). That men were chosen as the ideal travelers reveals once again the gendered phenomenon of travel (Leed, *The Mind*, 113).

54  Women of color scholars have called out traditional autoethnography for erasing "everyday political struggles," excluding women of color's experiences and voices, and being "overtly personal"—committed more to personal than to cultural transformation (Chawla, "Narratives," 106).

55  Chawla and Rodriguez, *Liminal*, 105–6. Traditional autoethnography focuses mostly on major life changes, deaths, or illnesses, which tends to "deprivilege stories about the ordinariness of living" (Chawla, "Narratives," 105–6).

56  Chawla, "Narratives," 110.

57  In sharing the intimate details of my life, I echo autoethnographer Carolyn Ellis in considering "personal narrative as a way to cope with personal issues and public troubles, as well as to provide companionship and comparative life experiences for those going through their own troubles," and "a way to write myself to understanding, insight and acceptance of whatever calamity fell my way" (Ellis, *Final*, 1, 3). That is, autoethnography is employed here as a method that not only can provide us with new understandings about the issue but can also help myself and others address the problems at hand, while simultaneously aiming to change the very culture that creates this issue to begin with. At its core, autoethnography "furnishes us with different perspectives on sociopolitical issues" (Chen, "Recollecting," 85).

58  Vidal-Ortiz, "On Being," 181.

59  Birkeland, *Making*, 30.

60  Yamamoto, *Masking*, 103.

61  Chawla, "Between Stories," 23. In crafting a narrator voice that invites the readers into its formation, I am also interested in finding out, as sociologist Arthur Frank points out, "what a listener *becomes* in the course of listening to the story" (Frank, *The Wounded*, 159). In this way, the self in transnational feminist autoethnography can never be a self-serving self because for as long as the story only tells the story of my own personal transformation, it "may pose no threat to the status quo. . . . The only way to change the condition of the world is by changing our knowledge of the world" (Chawla, "Narratives," 111).

62  Adams et al., *Autoethnography*, 90–91. I want to also note here that women of color scholars are often "caught between stories and theories—a liminal

intellectual space" (Chawla, "Between Stories," 9) and have to "navigate multiple discursive spaces, shifting between tactics in order to re-center power" and "shift between a storytelling approach *and* academic writing conventions" (H. Bhattacharya, *Narrating*, 7–8). Rather than forcing myself to choose one or the other, I follow these women of color scholars before me in embracing both. I do so to practice what I preach, which is to incorporate crossing in my research. In this way, transnational feminist autoethnography pays homage to feminist theorist M. Jacqui Alexander, who convinces us of the importance of both the crossing and the crossroads as "the space of convergence and endless possibility; the place where we put down and discard the unnecessary in order to pick up that which is necessary" (Alexander, *Pedagogies*, 8). It is where we can figure out "new ways of being and knowing" (Alexander, *Pedagogies*, 8).

Moreover, my wanting to claim a space in theory for women of color is also driven by the fact that I have often heard students complain about how certain writings (usually by women of color) that engage with deep theoretical thinking are "hard to read" (because our works have often appeared in the classroom simply to illustrate the hardship of our lived experiences and what it means to be a person of color in this world, but not as "theory") as a way to object to and dismiss them, and disqualify their inclusion in the classroom. However, these students would worship, emulate, and quote "complex academic" writings by celebrated theorists (often, by men and/or white scholars) whose inaccessible language/difficult-to-read texts are construed, instead, as "brilliant," and hence worth the time it takes to patiently work through their meanings.

63  Adams et al., *Autoethnography*, xvii.

64  I merge theories with stories in the hope that I may complicate the meanings and importance of story in autoethnography. My fascination with stories stems from my long-term training in the politics of representation, being aware that "representation is always oozing with power" (H. Bhattacharya, *Narrating*, 8). Story is indeed a means of representation and a way to craft and participate in discourse.

65  Keating and Bhattacharya, "Decolonizing," 524. Also see Anzaldúa, *Light*.

66  This means that my writing merges "self, culture, community, spirit, and theory" (K. Bhattacharya, "Autohistoria-teoría," 198).

67  Birkeland, *Making Place*, 30–31. The process of narration itself can be likened to "travelling into another landscape of meaning that is fictional" (Birkeland, *Making Place*, 106).

68  Story also makes legible the materiality and affectivity of experience. In this book, I use travel as a technology and a form of legibility in storytelling. Moreover, stories function to "traverse and organize places; they select and link them together; they make sentences and itineraries out of them. They are spatial trajectories" (de Certeau, "Spatial," 88). How we traverse these spaces also changes how we experience the space and tell the story, or, as women's studies and English professor Sidonie Smith points out, "Technologies of motion transform narratives

of travel" (Smith, *Moving*, xii). Walking, versus biking or other modes of exploring, shifts the story and theory that I tell (see chapter 5).

69 Chawla, "Narratives," 109–10.

70 I want to follow in the footsteps of autoethnography that exists in the space "between the orienting and disorienting story" (Gingrich-Philbrook, "Evaluating," 610).

71 Chawla, "Narratives," 109.

## CHAPTER 3. HOW CAN I PERCEIVE DIFFERENTLY?

1 Minimum-wage.org, "Costa Rica Minimum Wage Rate," www.minimum-wage. org. Last accessed April 19, 2022.

2 I intentionally keep the information vague so as to blur the identity of the owner, the retreat, the retreat facilitators, and anyone involved with the retreat.

3 US Department of State, "U.S. Relations."

4 To protect the privacy and identity of the participants and retreat organizers, and to be consistent with my method of autoethnography, I share only my own experiences at the retreat, and refer to other participants with nontraceable identifying information merely for contextual purposes.

5 I hope it is clear to the readers that by using the phrase "sexual magic," I do not slut-shame her.

6 For instance, pain studies scholars Louise Hide, Joanna Bourke, and Carmen Mangion argue that "pains are modes of perceptions: they are not the actual injury or noxious stimuli, but the way we evaluate the injury or stimuli" (Hide et al., "Introduction," 3). Similarly, as professor of clinical and experimental behavioral medicine Martin Diers explains, pain is "a *perceptual* phenomenon integrating and modulating several neuronal, psychological, and cultural processes and requires a conscious organism" (Diers, "Neuroimaging," 2, emphasis mine). Other scholars also point to how pain is not simply an emotion or an affect but rather "a mode of bodily perception" (Cohen et al., "Reconsidering," 4).

7 For philosopher Maurice Merleau-Ponty, perception is "our access to the truth"; it "establishes . . . our idea of the truth" (Merleau-Ponty, *Phenomenology*, xxx). By framing perception as our *access* to the truth, and something that allows us to grasp what the truth can be, he moves us away from considering perception as the truth itself (Merleau-Ponty, *Phenomenology*, xxx). For philosopher John Taber, because "perception is a means of knowledge, it should . . . function as an instrument that yields knowledge as its result" (Taber, *A Hindu*, 5). Moreover, perception is one of the sources of knowledge, a mode of approximating truth, and can be registered as "an epistemic modality" (Coseru, *Perceiving*, 155). Perception provides us with "cognitive access" (Davis and Thompson, "From," 648).

8 Gunning, "Arrogant," 198. It is important to note here that in feminist discourse, "arrogant perception" is often used to refer to white Western imperialist feminists

who have a white savior complex and fail to see the "other," often marginalized, third-world women, in their contexts. In my case, I use it to refer to myself, who centers the world around me and my victimhood subjectivity. Thus, although my use of the concept has a *meaning* similar to Gunning's, *whom* the concept refers to is not the same.

9  Gunning, "Arrogant," 202.

10  Gunning, "Arrogant," 199.

11  Gunning articulates it thus: "A key aspect of arrogant perception is the distance between 'me' and 'the other.' The 'I' as arrogant perceiver is a subject to myself with my own perceptions, motivations, and interests. The 'other,' in arrogant perception terms, is unlike me. The 'other' has no independent perceptions and interest but only those that I impose. Any evidence that the 'other' is organized around her own interests is evidence of defectiveness in the 'other.' The arrogant perceiver falsifies and oversimplifies" (Gunning, "Arrogant," 199).

12  Because the retreat leader has a book deal on her workshop activities—she explicitly wrote that everything in her book is copyrighted—I do not have the right to share the specific activities and prompts she designed for us and hence shy away from providing details. Instead, I focus on general activities and themes that commonly happen in other retreats as well: the transformation from a victim to a victor subjectivity.

13  Gunning, "Arrogant," 205, 213.

14  Philosopher Ali Mohsen discusses how this way of perceiving could cultivate "a standpoint epistemology that aims to empower authenticity through acknowledgement of the Other and promotes decolonized, intersectional habits of perceiving" (Mohsen, "Emotion," 244).

15  Mohsen, "Emotion," 83.

16  Foucault, "Docile," 240. The project of docile bodies is connected to the invention of the prison, where the supervision of what bodies need to do when, etc., happens. To read more about this, see Foucault, *Discipline*.

17  For more on the construction of gendered docile bodies, see Bartky, *Femininity*.

18  Foucault, "Docile," 240. This "docility" project is distinct in terms of (1) "the scale of the control." It works at the level of the individual body, and through "a subtle coercion" of the body's very mechanism and movements; (2) "the object of the control." This refers to what is being controlled, which is not only the "signifying elements" of the body but also the body's "internal organization" and forces; and (3) "the modality." Moreover, this "meticulous control of the operations of the body" is what he calls "discipline" (Foucault, "Docile," 240). It is this discipline that creates "subjected and practised bodies, 'docile' bodies" (Foucault, "Docile," 241).

19  To learn more about this concept of how inmates internalize that they are always under the surveillance of the prison guard, please read Foucault, *Discipline*.

20  Dreyfus and Rabinow, *Michel Foucault*, 152.

21  Mohsen points out, "We see here how perceiving the world that challenges the dominant paradigm is received as a hostile threat, and entire systems of control have been implemented to manage the emotions of the population" (Mohsen, "Emotion," 157).

22  Lysaught, "Docile," 390.

23  Lysaught, "Docile," 390.

24  When we tell stories through a particular discourse, it helps make sense of what happens to us. Once we perceive it to be the truth, we abide by it (when in fact it is only true or makes sense because we tell it from that specific discourse). We tend to not question or challenge what happens, or see "truth" itself as being produced "as a function of power" (Lysaught, "Docile," 391). As theologian M. Therese Lysaught argues, truth "points to the creation of knowledge as a function of power. Truth is a product of discursive practices understood to emerge only within a structure of rules, practices, and institutions that control the discourse and collaborate to establish a given claim as true. Knowledge shaped by discourses, empowered by institutions, and wielded through techniques and practices thus has the power to make itself true. Truth then is embodied and reproduced through 'rituals of truth,' practices shaped according to the rules of the discourse which then, not surprisingly, reinforce the truth-claims of the discourse" (Lysaught, "Docile," 391).

25  Alcoff, "Sexual," 454.

26  Mohsen, "Emotion," 153–54.

27  Alcoff, "Sexual," 454.

28  Mohsen, "Emotion," 147.

29  Engels, *The Origin*.

30  Firestone, *The Dialectic*, 131.

31  Think for a moment here of other forms of relationship that are nonmonogamous, such as polyamorous or open relationships.

32  Being docile thus signals that a person's "compliance" exists "within multiple networks of invisible, but always present, disciplinary powers" (Curtis, "Justice," 14).

33  Although in this chapter I use an example of how both arrogant and loving perceptions function as docile perception, docile perception does not always have to be either arrogant or loving. A perception is docile when it involves a disciplinary process (which we later internalize and normalize as our own) and reflects and supports dominant scripts and power.

34  The abbot and chief meditation master of Meetirigala Nissarana Vanaya Forest Monastery in Sri Lanka, Venerable Uda Eriyagama Dhammajīva Mahā Thero, stated that the Buddha likened "perception to a mirage" (Thero, *Anattalakkhana*, 31). He further stated that "a mirage lacks substance and gives an appearance which promises water. Our insatiable thirst chases after it with the promise of water, yet, the closer we come to it, the further we move

away from it. We neither reach the mirage nor reduce the distance" (Thero, *Anattalakkhana*, 31).

35   The nature of mirage is indeed impermanence. Thero puts it simply: "Perception is volatile; it evolves and changes" (Thero, *Anattalakkhana*, 28). How one perceives at a particular moment also depends on various elements: one's mood, "cognitive awareness . . . , interpretation . . . , behavioral dispositions . . . , cultural . . . and educational factors" (Bueno-Gómez, "Conceptualizing," 2).

It can also be influenced by a traumatic past and how a person processes it (Alcoff, "Sexual," 458). For instance, when a child is traumatized and they have not processed and transformed their experience, the working of their adult perception is based on the childhood perception that was "frozen" at the time of trauma (Tauber and van der Hal, "Transformation," 161). In other words, these adults function "with the perceptions of the wounded child" (Tauber and van der Hal, "Transformation," 162). Thus, a traumatic past can influence one's "variability of interpretations" (Alcoff, "Sexual," 458). When the exact same event happens to two different people, they may perceive and respond to it differently, on the basis of their past experiences. Psychotherapists Yvonne Tauber and Elisheva van der Hal, on the basis of their study of child survivors of the Holocaust (who were middle-aged at the time of research), found that how survivors "explained their traumas to themselves," both when the event happened and after the event, is crucial in determining the course of their lives (Tauber and van der Hal, 161). Those who "'parent' themselves by transforming their perceptions and subsequent life philosophy throughout their lives" were better able to cope with trauma (Tauber and van der Hal, "Transformation," 161). According to them, in dealing with painful and traumatizing events, it is important to work on the perception of these events to create new meanings that help people adjust after a major life disruption. In this way, they, too, highlight the important link between perception and one's experience of pain. Although I agree with Tauber and van der Hal, what I would like to emphasize here is how perception can still be unreliable and function as a mirage, even when we have healed our trauma.

36   Coseru, *Perceiving*, 190.

37   Insight Meditation South Bay, "Five Aggregates," 2; Coseru, *Perceiving*, 144. Moreover, the author of *Buddhist Psychology of Perception*, Ediriweera Saratchandra, points out that it is our unrelenting belief in our sensory apparatus as reliable and unchanging that is the problem. Saratchandra argues, "Sense-cognition is at the root of all the misery of this world. We perceive forms with our eyes, hear sounds with our ears, and get attached to them. But the things we get thus attached to are constantly changing, they disappear like bubbles at the slightest touch" (Saratchandra, *Buddhist*, 11). If we understand what we perceive based on our sensory apparatus as constantly changing, rather than permanent and truthful, then, as his logic goes, we may have a chance at releasing our misery.

38 There is a difference, according to philosopher Christian Coseru, between considering perception as fallible and calling it erroneous. Coseru clarifies, "Perception, while not infallible, is nevertheless a nonerroneous cognition. The sensory systems do not have the capacity to effect epistemic discriminations in terms of true or false, since we are warranted in accepting the contents of experience *qua* objects of sensory apprehension (hence the old adage: 'seeing is believing')" (Coseru, *Perceiving*, 183).

39 Coseru, *Perceiving*, 172.

40 Our limited range of perceptive possibilities can be influenced by the conditioning (or, to use Foucault's language, the "disciplining") of our perception. Our community, for instance, is one of the sites where we are conditioned to "perceive in similar ways" (Mohsen, "Emotion," 156). Philosopher Ali Mohsen argues, "The social milieu conditions our way of perceiving the world . . . and by habituating a particular way of perceiving we constitute the Self or Subject" (Mohsen, "Emotion," 102). Here, he recognizes that the Self is constructed out of *habituated perception*, and that this habituated perception is a result of social milieu conditioning. This conditioning of perception—the notion that environment, culture, communities, and social milieu determine the range of our perceptive possibilities—and how it serves the dominant ideology is what I call "docile perception."

41 Thero, *Anattalakkhana*, 33.

42 Thero, *Anattalakkhana*, 53.

43 Thero suggests, "When perception plays tricks, if you are prepared, mindfulness can cut through it. With the aid of mindfulness, one can transcend preference and judgment rooted in perception" (Thero, *Anattalakkhana*, 31).

44 Scott, "Experience," 26.

45 Scott, "Experience," 34.

46 I am not at all saying we should not buy sexy lingerie. I am saying that when I bought it excessively, without questioning what this practice of purchasing lingerie does to uphold ideologies of femininity, hetero/sexuality, etc., and to the point that I was sacrificing my overall financial wellness, it became problematic.

47 We also need to assess what access to power we have that can influence change. For instance, as an author, I can write; but others who are media practitioners can create media content that challenges the hegemony of monogamy, the trope of jealous lover, and the ageist/ableist/sexist/racist beauty standard. Policymaker and lawmakers can create policies that challenge sexist laws, etc.

48 By proposing docile perception, I aim to offer a different way of understanding perception, which is that when perception, or "experience," causes us pain, that does not necessarily happen because it is being "hijacked" as such (S. Siegel, *The Rationality*, 5).

CHAPTER 4. HOW CAN I WORK WITH MY BODY TO PROCESS PAIN?

1 Library of Congress, "Nepal."

2 Bansal et al., "Osho," 5.

3 Guerin, "Replacing," 44.

4 Wendorf and Yang, "Benefits," 273.

5 Kearney, "Narrating," 52.

6 Kearney, "Narrating," 61.

7 Bresin and Gordon, "Aggression," 402.

8 Bresin and Gordon, "Aggression," 401.

9 Cui, *Gendered*, 117.

10 June-Rodgers, "Bodily," 17.

11 Chen, "Recollecting," 108.

12 Bacon, "Narrative," 131. Stories also matter in feminist theorizing. Indeed, Claire Hemmings's book *Why Stories Matter: The Political Grammar of Feminist Theory* emphasizes the stakes that feminist scholars have in telling stories of feminism, especially ones that may be complicit in dominant narratives (i.e., global capitalism, hetero/sexism, racism, etc.) even as we attempt to challenge them. She thus calls for a different way of telling feminist stories that is more "ethically accountable" and "politically transformative" by paying attention to the citation system (i.e., she suggests we cite the institution rather than the author to highlight the institutional process of knowledge production), and to the affective politics of our narratives (Hemmings, *Why*, 2).

13 Ellis, "There," 727. Language and specific discourses (feminist discourses included) can be useful in helping us make sense of what happens and in shaping how we feel.

14 Bacon, "Narrative," 131; Kearney, "Narrating," 51.

15 I do want to make a methodological note here: I employ autoethnography in this chapter with a twist, albeit a theoretical one. Autoethnography believes in the power of narration and thus I work with my own personal stories. However, my argument stresses the importance of *nonstory* in processing pain and therein lies its paradox. As readers carefully and critically read my argument, I hope they can understand my point that it is not that I am arguing solely for nonstory but rather that we create spaces for nonstory to exist alongside stories, and value its usefulness for processing pain. I highlight nonstory to emphasize how in processing pain we need to register it at the level of the affective/body rather than *only* at the cognitive level per se. I want to add that being in Nepal, particularly in the specific meditation ashram that I visited, forced me to notice and hence make a distinction between what was foreign to me and what has become naturalized in my own life. It exposed me to new ways of being, living, and meditating. That the ashram called itself the "International Commune" and people from different countries such as China, Iran, India, Russia, United Arab Emirates, Australia, United States, Greece, and Nepal indeed were the ones I met and interacted with

also contributed to my thinking more carefully about language and where I am located within it—my relationship to it and to pain.

16  Satina and Hultgreen, "The Absent," 522.

17  Pagis, "Embodied," 265.

18  What is transformative or transcendental about this method is not simply the practice of catharsis, meditation, or the combined techniques per se that come one after the other. As Osho points out, "Whatever catharting one does, whatever integrating of the repressed, whatever acceptance of one's emotions would take place, ultimately *psychotherapy cannot lead to transformation*" (Amrito, "Rajneesh," 116, emphasis in original). Rather, it is "witnessing" and "transcending of the subject-object split" that allow for transcendence to happen—transcending pain is not simply about working through one's emotions (Amrito, "Rajneesh," 116). According to him, it is not only the first part of the meditation technique—catharsis—that transcended pain but also the second and third parts of meditation, which came after catharsis—the witnessing aspect of therapy—that leads to transformation.

19  Scarry, *The Body*, 4.

20  Frank, *The Wounded*, 28.

21  That is, via discourses, including feminist discourses.

22  Moss, "Defining," 489.

23  Orwell, *A Collection*, 171.

24  For more on this, see Derek Wolcott's work, and Devika Chawla's interpretation of Derek Walcott's text in "Poetic Arrivals and Departures: Bodying the Ethnographic Field in Verse."

25  Pfaelzer, "Tillie," 1.

26  Kabir, "Double," 158.

27  Alexander, *Pedagogies*, 316.

28  Silence, for instance, can be a survival mechanism for the oppressed group and a way to protect the integrity of the pain itself. For the oppressor, however, silence is never acceptable, as it reflects one's complicity in the power hierarchy. A more extended discussion on this issue can be read in Saraswati, *Pain Generation*, especially chapter 4, "Silence as Testimony in Margaret Cho's #12daysofrage."

29  For more on the limitations of voice and silence in articulating a feminist agency in the context of pain, see Saraswati, *Pain Generation*, 125–26. I recognize that words can at times function as a (double-edged) sword that can cut, divide, and hurt, even as they may heal at the same time. That is, words (others' or our own) may make the situation and the feeling worse. I thus offer the possibility of gibberish, which is not about being silent or having a voice but rather speaking without the story, in processing our pain.

CHAPTER 5. HOW CAN I PRACTICE FEMINIST ENCHANTMENT IN MY
EVERYDAY LIFE?

1 Enchantment as an embodied practice means that enchantment is something that we experience with our body (or register in the body). We can cultivate it through/with our body—we can train our body into experiencing enchantment.

2 In conceptualizing "feminist enchantment," I draw from enchantment theories and put them in a conversation with feminist theories. Enchantment began to receive serious consideration in academia, especially the social sciences, after sociologist Max Weber made a note about its opposite, disenchantment, in his 1918 lecture, translated into English as "Science as a Vocation." He wrote, "The fate of our times is characterized by rationalization and intellectualization and, above all, by the 'disenchantment of the world'" (Weber, "Science," 155). His lecture can be read as a call to find a new mode of being enchanted by the world without necessarily returning to religion. In 2006, George Levine published *Darwin Loves You: Natural Selection and the Re-enchantment of the World*, which convinces us how enchantment can exist in a secular world, where science still holds the power to shape how we understand what happens. Modernity need not be marred by disenchantment, but rather can remain "deeply entangled with magical and mythical thought" (Felski, *Uses*, 59). In this way, enchantment is powerful and important in our contemporary postmodern world not as the world's contrasting opposite but as its sustaining element. Here, enchantment is considered to be the glue that makes possible the connection among and between us, the modern world, and the sacred world.

3 Borenstein and Calin, *Fast*, 47.

4 Borenstein and Calin, *Fast*, 48.

5 Diers, "Neuroimaging," 2; Gudmannsdottir and Halldorsdottir, "Primacy," 318; Leder, "The Experiential," 454.

6 Leder, "The Experiential," 444; Gudmannsdottir and Halldorsdottir, "Primacy," 318.

7 Miles, "Pain," 43.

8 Apkarian et al., "Towards"; Ojala et al., "The Dominance," 141.

9 Diers, "Neuroimaging," 2.

10 Ojala et al., "The Dominance," 144.

11 These techniques work as they can change "the brain's processing of pain through an altered cerebral loop between pain signals, emotions, and cognitions, which leads to an increased access to executive regions for reappraisal of pain" (Diers, "Neuroimaging," 8).

12 My experiences in New Zealand and Nepal are discussed in different chapters.

13 Bennett, "The Enchanted," 4. Bennett also argues that enchantment can be experienced in "'secular' rather than sacred terms as a sensuous and joyful

immersion in the marvelous specificity of things" (referenced in Felski, *Uses*, 58). Bennett insists that enchantment "outlasted" the Enlightenment and still persists in today's world (Bennett, "The Enchanted," 1).

14  Bennett, *Enchantment*, 10; Felski, *Uses*, 58.

15  Felski, *Uses*, 54.

16  Felski, *Uses*, 54.

17  Felski, *Uses*, 76.

18  Bennett, "The Enchanted," 5.

19  Felski, *Uses*, 54.

20  As Levine points out, "moments of enchantment" matter because they "liberate us briefly from the pains of modern life" and "allow joy to enter and in so doing help us in our relations to the awfulness of so much that constitutes life around the globe" (Levine, *Darwin*, 14).

21  Felski, *Uses*, 54.

22  I frame forgetting in the way that queer theorist Jack Halberstam does, which is as a way to ideologically and politically subvert power and to break the pattern that reproduces the self as the authority that *knows*. This is to create a "rupture with the eternally self-generating present, a break with a self-authorizing past" (Halberstam, *The Queer*, 70). Halberstam argues that forgetting allows us to "produce an alternative mode of knowing, one that resists the positivism of memory projects" and can "be a useful tool for jamming the smooth operations of the normal and the ordinary" (Halberstam, *The Queer*, 69–70).

23  Halberstam, *The Queer*, 69–70.

24  Bennett, *Enchantment*, 5.

25  Manuel, "Transforming," 93.

26  By using the word "solely," I want to highlight that even though Lorde's articulation of the erotic frees us from its sexual connotations, my articulation of embodying the erotic still includes, although it is not limited to, these sexual meanings. In doing so, I turn to Alexander's framing of the erotic, which is that when women embrace our "erotic autonomy," make it women centered, and define it outside of our relationship with men, it can threaten the heterosexual family and even the nation that relies on the very reproduction of family/heterosexuality (Alexander, *Pedagogies*, 22). Nonetheless, similar to Lorde's, Alexander's articulation also expands the meanings of the erotic, as can be seen from her argument that "we need the erotic in our lives, in our analytic, political and pedagogic projects in ways that constitute the very fabric of our being" (Alexander, "Danger," 157). That is, when I "release" the erotic "from its intense and constrained pellet, it flows through and colors my life with a kind of energy that heightens and sensitizes and strengthens all of my experience" (Lorde, *Sister Outsider*). In this way, embodying the erotic and being spellbound share similar sensations and feelings of/in the body.

27  Lorde, *Sister Outsider*.

28 Young, "'Uses,'" 301. Women's and gender studies scholar Nikki Young offers us a critical insight into Lorde's notion of the erotic that may be helpful:

> This ongoing separation from one's self—one's body knowledge—is a result of a systematic maintenance of myopic modes of knowing. When we have been taught to suspect knowledges that are not socially (or religiously) sanctioned or institutionally derived, we deny the legitimacy of our deepest feelings as a way of knowing. . . . I employ Lorde's description of sensuality as an epistemological source in order to destabilize the polarization of mind and body. This destabilization is not only helpful in supporting a psychosomatic frame of knowing; it also encourages a new type of truth seeking that opens imaginative possibilities. (Young, "'Uses,'" 303)

29 It is to understand, as Young asserts, that "embodiment is a legitimate lens through which one can gain deeper understanding" (Young, "'Uses,'" 304–5).

30 Manuel, "Transforming," 87. As Manuel observes, "Enchantment is getting back to [one's] life and having a oneness, a connectedness to humanity" (Manuel, "Transforming," 120).

31 Bueno-Gómez, "Conceptualizing," 7–8.

32 Katz, "Pain," 59.

33 Svenaeus, "The Phenomenology," 121.

34 This means that as something "interior to the self" pain is "unshareable" and "inexpressible," making the sufferers feel alienated from themselves, in addition to from others (Leder, 453). Simultaneously, pain is also "threateningly exterior" as it "has the power to disintegrate our customary sense of relationship to others and our own embodiment" (Leder, "The Experiential," 454).

35 Katz, "Pain," 59.

36 Bennett, *Enchantment*, 10, emphasis mine.

37 Burlein and Orr, "Introduction," 15.

38 Lorde, *Sister Outsider*.

39 Levine, *Darwin*, 62.

40 Bennett, *Enchantment*, 5.

41 Revisit here Bennett's argument that "enchantment is something that we encounter, that hits us, but it is also a comportment that can be fostered through deliberate strategies. One of those strategies might be to give greater expression to the sense of play, another [is] to hone sensory receptivity to the marvelous specificity of things" (Bennett, *Enchantment*, 4).

42 Lugones, *Pilgrimages/Peregrinajes*, 83.

43 In some ways, this is similar to Bennett's notion of "an ethic of generosity toward others" (Bennett, *Enchantment*, 10).

44 Potter, "Tracing," 6.

45 In thinking of enchantment and linking it with power, feminism, and social justice, I am following in the footsteps of sociologists Julie Ham and Merina Sunuwar, who see "the potential of enchantment in social change efforts" (Ham

and Sunuwar, "Experiments," 2). In their analysis of Elpie Malicsi, a Filipino
domestic worker in Hong Kong, Ham and Sunuwar focus on Malicsi's creative
transformation in creating "intellectual and ethical disruptions for public
audiences" by way of her *Sustainable Sunday Couture*, featuring upcycled gowns
(Ham and Sunuwar, "Experiments," 1). They argue, "Any exploration of enchantment must be firmly embedded in an analysis of power and social difference,
particularly when understanding the effect of enchantment in social change
efforts" (Ham and Sunwar, "Experiments," 7). It is in this context that I see
enchantment as doing the feminist work of power disruption and pain
transformation.

46  Bird, *The Hawaiian*, xxv, 11, 21, 23, 161.
47  Naraindasa and Bastos, "Introduction," 6.
48  For example, people traveled to the Hathor temple at Dendera, Egypt, for healing
(Abouelata, "Travel," 121).
49  Kelley, *Excursions*, 136–37.
50  Kelley, *Excursions*, 136–37.
51  Dubrov, "Rational," 86.
52  Kinsley also notes that "travel offers not just greater insight, but a new dimension
of experience" (Kinsley, "Narrating," 72).
53  Julia Kristeva quoted in Kelley, *Excursions*, 21.
54  Kelley, *Excursions*, 133.
55  Kelley, *Excursions*, 23.
56  I also want to make visible how my eating habits are shaped by my habitus. That
is, Bourdieu points out that "whereas the working classes are more attentive to the
strength of the (male) body than its shape, and tend to go for products that are
both cheap and nutritious, the professions prefer products that are tasty, health-
giving, light and not fattening. Taste, a class culture turned into nature, that is,
*embodied*, helps to shape the class body" (Bourdieu, *Distinction*, 190).
57  Country Economy, "National."
58  See Tanya Golash-Boza, *Race*, 345. She also notes that "in this way, health
disparities can be linked directly to environmental racism: institutional policies
and practices that differentially affect the health outcomes or living conditions of
white and non-white communities are clear" (345).
59  I draw this argument from women's studies and English professor Sidonie Smith,
who has written extensively on this issue. She argues,

> Because vehicles of motion hold bodies in and to precise alignments with
> the ground, they fix and unfix distances—perceptual, temporal, and
> social—between the traveler and the landscape through which she moves.
> Propelled through space, the traveler becomes conscious of constantly
> shifting sensual data and impressions—sounds, sights, and smells. In this
> way the speed at which new impressions press upon the traveler's con-
> sciousness, the spatial distance that separates her from the source of those

impressions, and her perception of potential intimacy and disconnected-ness can expand and contract, contract and expand, depending upon the mode of transport. More broadly, modes of motion organize the entire sensorium differently and thus affect the conditions, the focalizing range, and the position of the perceiving subject, differentially connecting and disconnecting her to and from the terrain of travel, differentially organiz-ing her ways of negotiating unfamiliar territory, and differentially affecting systems of behavior. (Smith, *Moving*, 23)

60 As Bennett points out, "One of the ways that enchantment works is by slowing down or speeding up the usual tempo of something" (Bennett, *Enchantment*, 127).

61 Feminist phenomenologists remind us that we need to mark the body under examination, such as noting its gender, as gender defines how that body experi-ences the world and relates to other bodies (McWeeny, "The Feminist," 42).

62 Bennett, *Enchantment*, 6.

63 Gilles Deleuze and Felix Guattari quoted in Bennett, *Enchantment*, 6.

64 Bennett, *Enchantment*, 39.

65 Bennett, *Enchantment*, 40.

66 Bennett, *Enchantment*, 40.

67 Bennett, "The Enchanted," 6.

68 Chawla, "Tracing Home's Habits," 4.

69 Bosnak, *Embodiment*, 25.

70 Bennett, *Enchantment*, 10. I want to clarify that here, I don't take it to mean that we look for the beauty in life so we can forget or dismiss pain but rather that we look for the beauty in the pain experience itself. That way, we don't dismiss and deny our pain.

71 Bennett, "The Enchanted," 8.

72 Bennett, "The Enchanted," 8; Weber, "Science," 139.

73 In English professor Susan Roberson's words, "When one moves through space, travels, relocates, then the 'who I am' undergoes some kind of transformation: the 'ecology of the self' is restructured with a change in the environment" (Roberson, *Defining*, xvii). Similarly, communications and rhetoric studies professor Amardo Rodriguez argues that "our bodies and ecologies shape how we perceive and make sense of things. When our bodies and ecologies change, how we perceive and make sense of things changes. There is no understanding of anything that is outside and separate from our bodies and ecologies" (Rodriguez, "The Exile Narratives," 112). Rodriguez's argument is also important in understanding the context (in this case, the body and ecology) of perception—see chapter 3.

74 On this matter, Bourdieu argues, "The habitus is not only a structuring structure, which organizes practices and the perception of practices, but also a structured structure: the principle of division into logical classes which organizes the perception of the social world is itself the product of internalization of the division into social classes" (Bourdieu, *Distinction*, 170).

75 If "life-styles are thus the systematic products of habitus, which, perceived in their mutual relations through the schemes of the habitus, become sign systems that are socially qualified" (Bourdieu, *Distinction*, 172), the new habitual body is not about the production of lifestyles. It is about encouraging the body to continually change, to take a new route in our walking, to be repetitive with a twist, and to find new ways to be enchanted.

## CHAPTER 6. HOW DOES WHERE I LIVE MATTER TO MY PAIN?

1 World Economic Forum, "New Zealand."
2 BBC News, "Iceland."
3 It is worthy of note that in Indonesia, news articles reported that the number of cases and deaths may not be counted properly and limited access to testing may further skew these numbers.
4 Fowers and Wan, "A Third."
5 Biesecker and Winterfeld, "Notion," 283.
6 Berns, "Liberalism," 146.
7 Biesecker and Winterfeld, "Notion," 284.
8 Puwar and Pateman, "Interview," 123; Pateman, *The Sexual*.
9 C. Mills, *The Racial*, 13–14.
10 Biesecker and Winterfeld, "Notion," 286.
11 Mohsen, "Emotion," 160.
12 Walsh, "Feminism," 835.
13 An article in *Ms.* magazine argues that we need to elect women if we want a happier country (Eisler and Baker, "Want to Make"). Certainly, as Eisler and Baker also show in their article, what we need is not only women officials but also gendered politics that are centered around people's well-being.
14 See Biesecker and Winterfeld, "Notion," 284.
15 Biesecker and Winterfeld, "Notion," 288; McRobbie, "Top," 730.
16 Other feminist theorists have also "challenged this elimination of affect from the realm of the political. . . . Affect . . . is . . . viewed by masculinist political theory as antagonistic to the demands of civilization and to the requirements of justice" (Stewart-Steinberg, "Girls," 26).
17 See Mohsen, "Emotion," 157, 210, 247.
18 Mohsen, "Emotion," 157.
19 For instance, although boys are often told not to cry—"boys don't cry"—as doing so would undermine their masculinity (remember, emotion is the domain of the feminine), during the nomination process and hearing related to his sexual misconduct, Bret Kavanaugh *did* express his emotions full-on, even tearing up as he declared his innocence. His display of emotions, particularly as he was choking up as he was sharing the story about how during her bedtime, his ten-year-old daughter wanted to pray for the woman who made the allegation, is seen as extraordinary—it framed him as a good Catholic father. It supported his claim,

"That's not who I am. It is not who I was. I am innocent of this charge." The result: he ascended to the US Supreme Court nonetheless.

On the contrary, a study reported that Hillary Clinton's failure to rise to the presidency was related to how Americans perceived her as being too emotional to lead—her being too emotional is related to her being a woman, that is, her gender, and not necessarily to a particular event or evidence. (For news coverage on this, see Emily Tillett, "Some Americans Still Doubt Women's Emotional Suitability for Politics, according to Study.") Thus, the gender of the politician and the context of the event matter: emotions can be permissible and deployed as an instrument of power by some politicians to serve and protect their interests, but not by or for others. For pointing out this insightful analysis, I would like to thank the anonymous reviewer.

20  Williams, *The Pursuit*, 38.

21  Garland-Thomson, "Feminist," 1557.

22  National Institute of Mental Health, "Statistics," https://www.nimh.nih.gov. Last accessed April 18, 2022.

23  Rousseau, *The Social*.

24  Keating, "Framing," 131.

25  Rousseau, *The Social*.

26  I am following in the footsteps of feminist theorist Angela McRobbie in her theorizing the concept "new sexual contract" as a cultural contract (McRobbie, "Top," 734–35).

27  Roy, "New Zealand."

28  Community and Public Health Te Mana Ora, "Mental Health."

29  Roy, "New Zealand."

30  Tikkanen et al., "International . . . New Zealand." Also see Te Kāwanatanga o Aotearoa New Zealand Government, "Getting Publicly Funded Health Services."

31  Tikkanen et al., "International . . . New Zealand."

32  New Zealand Now, "Healthcare."

33  Tikkanen et al., "International . . . New Zealand."

34  Tikkanen et al., "International . . . New Zealand."

35  Ardern, "Prime Minister."

36  People who live in socioeconomically deprived areas were "2.5 times more likely to experience psychological distress as people living in the least deprived areas." See Community and Public Health Te Mana Ora, "Mental Health."

37  New Zealand Now, "Paying."

38  Tikkanen et al., "International . . . New Zealand."

39  Ardern, "Prime Minister."

40  Mariskind, "Good," 15.

41  Defined as "the Māori tradition of children being raised by someone other than their birth parents." See here, Te Kāwanatanga o Aotearoa New Zealand Government, "Whāngai."

42  Employment New Zealand, "Types."

43  Mariskind, "Good," 18.

44  See Mariskind, "Good," 18. Since the 1980s, the neoliberal governance in New Zealand has increasingly relied on privatization, flexible employment, and decreased support of welfare. Under the neoliberal social contract, citizens are constructed as "active individuals" through "the exercise of personal choice"; and the gendered notion of citizen subjectivity shifts from citizen-mothers (unpaid) to citizen-workers (paid). As "citizen-workers," women's key responsibility is to be paid workers (rather than to be mothers whose work is unpaid) and this decision to be paid workers must be seen as a *personal* choice. Hence, "Mothers are required to be employees first and carers only secondarily" (Mariskind, "Good," 15). Mariskind's argument is especially insightful in that it helps us see how through this policy, the New Zealand government makes possible "a version of the social contract that both enables and resists responsibilised neoliberal subjectivities" (Mariskind, "Good," 14).

45  New Zealand Immigration, "Live."

46  Graham-McLay, "Under Pressure."

47  ABC/AP, "Jacinda Ardern."

48  Asafo, "'Kindness.'"

49  Sjúkratryggingar Íslands, "Payment."

50  Iceland Review, "In Focus."

51  Iceland Review, "In Focus."

52  Iceland Review, "In Focus."

53  Iceland Review, "In Focus."

54  Work in Iceland, "Maternity and Paternity Leave," https://work.iceland.is. Last accessed June 12, 2022.

55  Work in Iceland, "Maternity."

56  Work in Iceland, "Maternity."

57  BBC News, "Iceland."

58  Heleniak and Sigurjonsdottir, "Once Homogenous."

59  Útlendingastofnun: The Directorate of Immigration, "Service."

60  Útlendingastofnun: The Directorate of Immigration, "Service."

61  Útlendingastofnun: The Directorate of Immigration, "Service."

62  See the website of W.O.M.E.N in Iceland, http://womeniniceland.is/en. Last accessed April 18, 2022.

63  As theorist Shaka McGlotten suggests, "Personhood is not necessarily constituted by what one does, but by how one feels, and by the ways one names those feelings (or doesn't) and puts them into relationship (or doesn't) with larger social histories of difference or national belonging. Affect allows you to recognize when you are accepted or simply being tolerated" (referenced in Williams, *The Pursuit*, 38). It is thus important, in the articulation of one's citizenship and national belonging, that we incorporate emotion as well.

64 Rajiva, "'Better,'" 21.
65 Kharisma, "3 Hal Yang."
66 Humas, "Per 1 Mei."
67 Gerintya, "Statistik." Also see WHO website, "Mental Health Workers Data by Country." Based on more recent data from the Ministry of Health (Kementrian Kesehatan), in 2021, the ratio is one psychiatrist to 250,000 people (see Rokom, "Kemenkes").
68 Sebayang, et al., "Less Than 1,000."
69 DaffaDeliandra, "Indonesia."
70 DaffaDeliandra, "Indonesia."
71 DaffaDeliandra, "Indonesia." I also use data from the 2017 Global Health Data Exchange.
72 Tikkanen et al., "International . . . United States."
73 Tikkanen et al., "International . . . United States."
74 Tikkanen et al., "International . . . United States."
75 Because healthcare is not affordable for all, it is not a surprise that "people with higher incomes live longer, healthier lives" (Golash-Boza, *Race*, 322).
76 Tikkanen et al., "International . . . United States."
77 Tikkanen et al., "International . . . United States."
78 Golash-Boza, *Race*, 333.
79 Tikkanen et al., "International . . . United States."
80 Tikkanen et al., "International . . . United States."
81 National Institute of Mental Health, "Any Anxiety," www.nimh.nih.gov. Last accessed June 12, 2022.
82 National Institute of Mental Health, "Any Anxiety."
83 Anxiety and Depression Association of America, "Facts & Statistics."
84 National Institute of Mental Health, "Major Depression," www.nimh.nih.gov. Last accessed June 12, 2022.
85 National Institute of Mental Health, "Any Anxiety."
86 National Institute of Mental Health, "Post-Traumatic."
87 National Institute of Mental Health, "Major Depression."
88 The complete list of the forty-one countries can be viewed here: Livingston and Thomas, "Among 41 Countries."
89 Globalization Partners, "Indonesia."
90 US Citizenship and Immigration Services, "Find Help."
91 Golash-Boza, *Race*, 339.
92 World Happiness Report, "World Happiness Report 2017," March 20, 2017, https://worldhappiness.report.
93 World Happiness Report, "World Happiness."
94 Huffington, "Politics."
95 Castor, *Spiritual*, 6.

96 Think here also of Aihwa Ong's work in *Flexible Citizenship*, which Castor builds on. What I appreciate about Castor's theorization of spiritual citizenship is how it allows us to "decente[r] . . . U.S. racial systems" by "open[ing] up a space for a differentiated blackness, one intimately tied to a larger transnational community of the African diaspora" (Castor, *Spiritual*, 68).

97 Cvetkovich, *Depression*, 1.

98 Chen, "Recollecting," 108.

99 Livingston, "The Social," 187.

## CHAPTER 7. HOME(OSTASIS) IS WHERE THE HEART IS . . . HEALED

1 Ahmed, *Queer Phenomenology*, 9.

2 Fitzpatrick, "What She Carries," 13.

3 Anzaldúa, *Borderlands/La Frontera*.

4 Abdurraqib, "A House," 29; Blunt and Varley, "Introduction," 3; Chawla, *Home*, 27; Etemaddar et al., "Experiencing," 506; Nititham, *Making*, 40; Tsolidis, "Memories," 417; Walters, *At Home*, ix; Facio, "Spirit," 60.

5 Chawla and Jones, "Introduction," xi; Dunn, "Carrying," 70; hooks, *Yearning*, 148; Ismael and Ismael, "Between," 204; Mallet, "Understanding," 62.

6 Anderson, "Musing," 18; Wyatt and Wyatt, "(Be)Coming," 32.

7 Roberson, *Defining*, xvi.

8 Bhabha, "The World," 141.

9 Belcourt, *This Wound*, 34.

10 Buitelaar and Stock, "Making," 165.

11 Etemaddar et al., "Experiencing," 516.

12 Etemaddar et al., "Experiencing," 514.

13 Etemaddar et al., "Experiencing," 512; Buitelaar and Stock, "Making," 166.

14 Dunn, "Carrying," 89.

15 Mulla, *The Violence*, 177.

16 hooks, *Yearning*, 49.

17 For anthropologist James Clifford and literary historian Paul Fussell, home is imagined as a space where the "consolidation of the Self enabled by the encounter with the 'Other'" happens (Grewal, *Home*, 6). This is how home is distinguished from "abroad." For me, home becomes a place where I and the home itself come undone, over and over again. There is no distinction between here and there.

18 Kaplan, *Questions*, 194.

19 Anzaldúa, *Borderlands*, 21.

20 Jussawalla, "South," 19.

21 Friedman, "Bodies," 191.

22 Chawla, *Home*, 26.

23 Home can even be understood "as movement and motion rather than rootedness and stability" (Chawla, *Home*, 31).

24  Walters, *At Home*, 132.

25  An understanding of "home" that is closest to healing is "homewell." This concept refers to feeling "rooted, nurtured, aligned, synchronized, whole, plugged in and flowing. When you have *homewell*, what is essential—hearth, home, love, community, belonging, memory, creativity—is with you" (Knopp, "Household," 725).

26  Winkelman and Dubisch, "Introduction," xxvi.

27  Frankel, "Repentance," 815.

28  Scholar Rafi Nets-Zehngut points out that people who have a "self-healing personality" are "inclined to more protect personal health and to heal relatively quickly from illness" (Nets-Zehngut, "Collective," 246). Such a personality is a result of "genetics, personal habits, and emotional responses" as well as "psychological characteristics" (246). A study by Tedeschi, Park, and Calhoun shows that between 40 and 60 percent of trauma survivors heal themselves, "without external professional aid" (referenced in Nets-Zehngut, "Collective," 247).

29  Britannica, "Homeostasis."

30  Ahmed, *The Promise*, 11.

31  Macallister et al., "Exploring," 128.

32  Khattak, "Violence," 123.

33  Espiritu, *Home*; Gupta and Ferguson, referenced in Kim, "Digital Diaspora," 58.

34  Khattak, "Violence," 123.

35  Escandell and Tapias, "Transnational," 418–19.

# BIBLIOGRAPHY

ABC/AP. "Jacinda Ardern: What We Can Expect under New Zealand's New PM." Australian Broadcasting Company, October 20, 2017. www.abc.net.au.

Abdurraqib, Samaa. "A House Is Not Always a Home: Women's Writing of Home/Lands and Diaspora." PhD diss., University of Wisconsin, 2010.

Abouelata, Mohamed. "Travel to the Healing Centers in the Egyptian Temples: The Prototype of the Modern Medical Tourism." *Egyptian Journal of Archaeological and Restoration Studies* 8, no. 2 (2018): 121–32.

Adams, Tony, Stacy Jones, and Carolyn Ellis. *Autoethnography.* Oxford University Press, 2014.

Ahmed, Sara. "The Contingency of Pain." *Parallax* 8, no. 1 (2002): 17–34.

———. *The Cultural Politics of Emotion.* Edinburgh University Press, 2014.

———. *The Promise of Happiness.* Duke University Press, 2010.

———. *Queer Phenomenology: Orientations, Objects, Others.* Duke University Press, 2006.

Alacovska, Ana. "Genre Anxiety: Women Travel Writers' Experience of Work." *Sociological Review* 63, no. S1 (2015): 128–43.

Alcoff, Linda. "Sexual Violations and the Question of Experience." *New Literary History* 45, no. 3 (2014): 445–62.

Alexander, M. Jacqui. "Danger and Desire: Crossings Are Never Undertaken All at Once or Once and for All." *Small Axe* 24 (October 2007): 154–66.

———. *Pedagogies of Crossing: Meditations on Feminism, Sexual Politics, Memory, and the Sacred.* Duke University Press, 2005.

Alù, Giorgia. "Fabricating Home: Performances of Belonging and Domesticity in Contemporary Women's Travel Writing in English about Italy." *Studies in Travel Writing* 14, no. 3 (2010): 285–302.

Amrito, Swami Deva. "Rajneesh Therapy." *Journal of Humanistic Psychology* 24, no. 1 (1984): 115–18.

Anderson, Myrdene. "Musing on Nomadism: Being and Becoming at Home on the Reindeer Range." In *Stories of Home: Place, Identity, Exile*, edited by Devika Chawla and Stacy Holman Jones, 17–30. Lexington Books, 2015.

Anxiety and Depression Association of America. "Facts & Statistics." ADAA website. Last accessed April 18, 2022. https://adaa.org.

Anzaldúa, Gloria. *Borderlands/La Frontera: The New Mestiza.* Aunt Lute Books, 1987.

———. *Interviews/Entrevistas.* Edited by AnaLouise Keating. Routledge, 2000.

——. *Light in the Dark/Luz en lo Oscuro: Rewriting Identity, Spirituality, Reality.* Edited by AnaLouise Keating. Duke University Press, 2015.

Apkarian, A. Vania, et al. "Towards a Theory of Chronic Pain." *Progress in Neurobiology* 87, no. 2 (2009): 81–97.

Ardern, Jacinda. "Prime Minister Jacinda Ardern's Wellbeing Budget Speech." New Zealand Government, May 30, 2019. www.beehive.govt.nz.

Asafo, Dylan. "'Kindness' as Violence in the Settler-Colonial State of New Zealand." *Knowledge Culture* 9, no. 3 (2021): 39–53.

Bacon, Eugen. "Narrative and Narrative Strategies to Explore Trauma: 'Up Close from Afar'—an African Migrant's Story." *Australasian Review of African Studies* 37, no. 2 (2016): 129–46.

Bansal, Anuj, et al. "Osho Dynamic Meditation's Effect on Serum Cortisol Level." *Journal of Clinical and Diagnostic Research* 10, no. 11 (2016), https://doi.org/10.7860/JCDR/2016/23492.8827.

Bardwell-Jones, Celia. "Travel, Home, and the Space Between: A Feminist Pragmatist Approach to Transnational Identities." PhD diss., University of Oregon, 2007.

Bartky, Sandra. *Femininity and Domination: Studies in the Phenomenology of Oppression.* Routledge, 1990.

BBC News. "Iceland Puts Well-Being ahead of GDP in Budget." BBC, December 3, 2019. www.bbc.com.

Belcourt, Billy-Ray. *This Wound Is a World.* University of Minnesota Press, 2019.

Bennett, Jane. "The Enchanted World of Modernity: Paracelsus, Kant, and Deleuze." *Journal for Cultural Research* 1, no. 1 (1997): 1–28.

——. *The Enchantment of Modern Life: Attachments, Crossings, and Ethics.* Princeton University Press, 2001.

Berns, Sandra. "Liberalism and the Privatised Family: The Legacy of Rousseau." *Res Publica* 11 (2005): 125–55.

Bhabha, Homi. "The World and the Home." *Social Text* 141, no. 31/32 (1992): 141–53.

Bhattacharya, Himika. *Narrating Love and Violence.* Rutgers University Press, 2017.

Bhattacharya, Kakali. "Autohistoria-teoría: Merging Self, Culture, Community, Spirit, and Theory." *Journal of Autoethnography* 1, no. 2 (2020): 198–202.

Biesecker, Adelheid, and Uta von Winterfeld. "Notion of Multiple Crisis and Feminist Perspectives on Social Contract." *Gender, Work, and Organization* 25, no. 3 (2018): 279–93.

Bird, Isabella. *The Hawaiian Archipelago: Six Months among the Palm Groves, Coral Reefs, and Volcanoes of the Sandwich Islands.* 1890. Charles E. Tuttle Company, 1974.

Birkeland, Inger. *Making Place, Making Self: Travel, Subjectivity, and Sexual Difference.* Ashgate, 2005.

Blunt, Alison, and Ann Varley. "Introduction: Geographies of Home." *Cultural Geographies* 11 (2004): 3–6.

Bochner, Arthur. "Putting Meanings into Motion: Autoethnography's Existential Calling." In *Handbook of Autoethnography*, edited by Stacy Holman Jones, Tony E. Adams, and Carolyn Ellis, 50–56. 2013. Routledge, 2016.

Borenstein, David, and Andei Calin. *Fast Facts: Low Back Pain*. Health Press Limited, 2012.

Bosnak, Robert. *Embodiment: Creative Imagination in Medicine, Art, and Travel*. Routledge, 2008.

Bost, Suzanne. "Gloria Anzaldúa's Mestiza Pain: Mexican Sacrifice, Chicana Embodiment, and Feminist Politics." *Aztlán* 30, no. 2 (2005): 5–34.

Bourdieu, Pierre. *Distinction: A Social Critique of the Judgment of Taste*. Translated by Richard Nice. 1979. Routledge and Kegan Paul, 1984.

Brabant, Isabelle. "Reflections on Pain in Childbirth." In *When Pain Strikes*, edited by Bill Burns, Cathy Busby, and Kim Sawchuk, 47–55. University of Minnesota Press, 1999.

Brennan, Teresa. *The Transmission of Affect*. Cornell University Press, 2004.

Bresin, Konrad, and Kathryn Gordon. "Aggression as Affect Regulation: Extending Catharsis Theory to Evaluate Aggression and Experiential Anger in the Laboratory and Daily Life." *Journal of Social and Clinical Psychology* 32, no. 4 (2013): 400–423.

Britannica. "Homeostasis." Britannica website. Last accessed March 23, 2022. www.britannica.com.

Brown, Wendy. *States of Injury*. Princeton University Press, 1995.

Bueno-Gómez, Noelia. "Conceptualizing Suffering and Pain." *Philosophy, Ethics, and Humanities in Medicine* 12, no. 7 (2017), https://doi.org/10.1186/s13010-017-0049-5.

Buitelaar, Marjo, and Femke Stock. "Making Homes in Turbulent Times: Moroccan-Dutch Muslims Contesting Dominant Discourses of Belonging." In *Muslim Diaspora in the West: Negotiating Gender, Home, and Belonging*, edited by Haideh Moghissi and Halleh Ghorashi, 163–79. Ashgate, 2010.

Burlein, Ann, and Jackie Orr. "Introduction: The Practice of Enchantment; Strange Allures." *Women's Studies Quarterly* 40, no. 3/4 (2012): 13–23.

Burns, Bill, Cathy Busby, and Kim Sawchuk, eds. *When Pain Strikes*. University of Minnesota Press, 1999.

Butler, Pamela W. "Global Chicks: The Politics of Travel in Twenty–first-century Feminisms." PhD diss., University of Minnesota, 2011.

Castor, N. Fadeke. *Spiritual Citizenship: Transnational Pathways from Black Power to Ifá in Trinidad*. Duke University Press, 2017.

Chawla, Devika. "Between Stories and Theories: Embodiments, Disembodiments, and Other Struggles." *Storytelling, Self, Society: An Interdisciplinary Journal of Storytelling Studies* 3, no. 1 (Winter 2007): 16–30.

———. *Home, Uprooted: Oral Histories of India's Partition*. Fordham University Press, 2014.

———. "Narratives on Longing, Being, and Knowing: Envisioning a Writing Epistemology." In *Liminal Traces: Storying, Performing, and Embodying Postcoloniality*, edited by Devika Chawla and Amardo Rodriguez, 97–111. Sense Publishers, 2011.

————. "Poetic Arrivals and Departures: Bodying the Ethnographic Field in Verse." *Forum: Qualitative Social Research* 9, no. 2 (2008), http://nbn-resolving.de/urn:nbn:de:0114-fqs0802248.

————. "Tracing Home's Habits: Affective Rhythms." In *Stories of Home: Place, Identity, Exile*, edited by Devika Chawla and Stacy Holman Jones, 3–16. Lexington Books, 2015.

Chawla, Devika, and Ahmet Atay. "Introduction: Decolonizing Autoethnography." *Cultural Studies ↔ Critical Methodologies* 18, no. 1 (2018): 3–8.

Chawla, Devika, and Stacy Holman Jones. "Introduction." In *Stories of Home: Place, Identity, Exile*, edited by Devika Chawla and Stacy Holman Jones, xi–xxiii. Lexington Books, 2015.

Chawla, Devika, and Amardo Rodriguez. *Liminal Traces: Storying, Performing, and Embodying Postcoloniality*. Sense Publishers, 2011.

Chen, Guan-Rong. "Recollecting Memory, Reviewing History: Trauma in Asian North American Literature." PhD diss., University of Texas, 2008.

Clifford, James. *Routes: Travel and Translation in the Late Twentieth Century*. Harvard University Press 1997.

Clough, Patricia. "Autotelecommunication and Autoethnography: A Reading of Carolyn Ellis's *Final Negotiations*." *Sociological Quarterly* 38, no. 1 (1997): 95–110.

Cohen, Milton, et al. "Reconsidering the International Association for the Study of Pain Definition of Pain." *Pain Reports* (2018): 1–7.

Community & Public Health Te Mana Ora. "Mental Health and Illness." Community & Public Health Te Mana Ora website. Last accessed March 23, 2022. www.cph.co.nz.

Coseru, Christian. *Perceiving Reality: Consciousness, Intentionality, and Cognition in Buddhist Philosophy*. Oxford University Press, 2012.

Country Economy. "National Minimum Wage—Montenegro." Country Economy website. Last accessed March 23, 2022. https://countryeconomy.com.

Crane, Brent. "For a More Creative Brain, Travel." *Atlantic*, March 31, 2015. www.theatlantic.com.

Cui, Shuqin. *Gendered Bodies: Toward a Women's Visual Art in Contemporary China*. University of Hawai'i Press, 2016.

Curtis, Carl. "Justice, Punishment, and Docile Bodies: Michel Foucault and the Fiction of Franz Kafka." PhD diss., Florida State University, 2010.

Cvetkovich, Ann. *Depression: A Public Feeling*. Duke University Press, 2012.

DaffaDeliandra, Muhammad. "Indonesia Darurat Kesehatan Mental?" *Kompasiana*, December 27, 2019. www.kompasiana.com.

Davis, Jake H., and Evan Thompson. "From the Five Aggregates to Phenomenal Consciousness: Towards a Cross-Cultural Cognitive Science." In *A Companion to Buddhist Philosophy*, edited by Steven M. Emmanuel, 165–87. Wiley, 2013.

De Certeau, Michel. "Spatial Stories." *Defining Travel: Diverse Visions*, edited by Susan Roberson, 88–104. University Press of Mississippi, 2001.

De Mul, Sarah. *Colonial Memory: Contemporary Women's Travel Writing in Britain and the Netherlands*. Amsterdam University Press, 2011.

Diers, Martin. "Neuroimaging the Pain Network—Implications for Treatment." *Best Practice and Research Clinical Rheumatology* 33, no. 3 (June 2019), https://doi.org/10.1016/j.berh.2019.05.003.

Dollard, John, et al. *Frustration and Aggression*. Yale University Press, 1939.

Dreyfus, Hubert, and Paul Rabinow. *Michel Foucault: Beyond Structuralism and Hermeneutics*. University of Chicago Press, 1983.

Dubrov, Andrew. "Rational Enchantment: On the Travel Writings of Cendrars, Leiris, and Michaux." PhD diss., New York University, 2017.

Dunn, Carolyn. "Carrying the Fire Home: Performing Nation, Identity, Indigenous Diaspora, and Home in the Poems, Songs, and Performances of Arigon Starr, Joy Harjo, and Gayle Ross." PhD diss., University of Southern California, 2010.

Eisler, Riane, and Robyn Baker. "Want to Make Your Country Happier? Elect Women." *Ms.*, July 19, 2021. https://msmagazine.com.

Ellis, Carolyn. *Final Negotiations: A Story of Love, Loss, and Chronic Illness*. Temple University Press, 2018.

———. "Preface: Carrying the Torch for Autoethnography." In *Handbook of Autoethnography*, edited by Stacy Holman Jones, Tony E. Adams, and Carolyn Ellis, 9–12. 2013. Routledge London, 2016.

———. "'There Are Survivors': Telling a Story of Sudden Death." *Sociological Quarterly* 34, no. 4 (1993): 711–30.

Ellis, Carolyn, Tony Adams, and Arthur Bochner. "Autoethnography: An Overview." *Qualitative Social Research* 12, no. 1 (2011), http://nbnresolving.de/urn:nbn:de:0114-fqs1101108.

Employment New Zealand. "Types of Parental Leave." Employment New Zealand website. Last accessed March 23, 2022. www.employment.govt.nz.

Engels, Friedrich. *The Origin of the Family, Private Property, and the State*. 1884. Electric Book, 2001.

Escandell, Xavier, and Maria Tapias. "Transnational Lives, Travelling Emotions, and Idioms of Distress among Bolivian Migrants in Spain." *Journal of Ethnic and Migration Studies* 36, no. 3 (2010): 407–23.

Espiritu, Yen Le. *Home Bound: Filipino American Lives across Cultures, Communities, and Countries*. University of California Press, 2003.

Etemaddar, Mitra, et al. "Experiencing 'Moments of Home' through Diaspora Tourism and Travel." *Tourism Geographies* 18, no. 5 (2016): 503–19.

Euben, Roxanne. *Journeys to the Other Shore: Muslim and Western Travelers in Search of Knowledge*. Princeton University Press, 2006.

Facio, Elisa. "Spirit Journey: 'Home' as a Site for Healing and Transformation." In *Fleshing the Spirit: Spirituality and Activism in Chicana, Latina, and Indigenous Women's Lives*, edited by Elisa Facio and Irene Lara, 59–72. University of Arizona Press, 2014.

Felski, Rita. *Uses of Literature*. Wiley-Blackwell, 2008.

Firestone, Shulamith. *The Dialectic of Sex: The Case for Feminist Revolution*. Farrar, Straus and Giroux, 1970.

Fitzpatrick, Kristin. "What She Carries with Her: Gender and American National Identity in Nineteenth-Century Women's Travel Narratives." PhD diss., University of Washington, 1999.

Forte, Jeanie. "Focus on the Body: Pain, Praxis, and Pleasure in Feminist Performance." *Critical Theory and Performance*, edited by Janelle Reinelt and Joseph Roach, 248–62. University of Michigan Press, 1992.

Foucault, Michel. *Discipline and Punish: The Birth of the Prison*. Vintage Books, 1979.

———. "Docile Bodies." *Theatre and Performance Design: A Reader in Scenography*, edited by Jane Collins and Andrew Nisbet, 239–42. Routledge, 2010.

Fowers, Alyssa, and William Wan. "A Third of Americans Now Show Signs of Clinical Anxiety or Depression, Census Bureau Finds amid Coronavirus Pandemic." *Washington Post*, May 26, 2020. www.washingtonpost.com.

Frank, Arthur. *The Wounded Storyteller: Body, Illness, and Ethics*. 2nd ed. University of Chicago Press, 1995.

Frankel, Estelle. "Repentance, Psychotherapy, and Healing through a Jewish Lens." *American Behavioral Scientist* 41 (1998): 814–33.

Franklin, Adrian, and Mike Crang. "The Trouble with Tourism and Travel Theory?" *Tourist Studies* 1, no. 1 (2001): 5–22.

Friedman, Susan. "Bodies on the Move: A Poetics of Home and Diaspora." *Tulsa Studies in Women's Literature* 23, no. 2 (2004): 189–212.

Garland-Thomson, Rosemarie. "Feminist Disability Studies." *Signs: Journal of Women in Culture and Society* 30, no. 2 (2005): 1557–87.

Gerintya, Scholastica. "Statistik Bunuh Diri dan Darurat Kesehatan Mental." *Tirto.id*, March 18, 2017. https://tirto.id.

Gilbert, Elizabeth. *Eat, Pray, Love*. Riverhead Books, 2007.

Gilmore, Leigh. "Agency without Mastery: Chronic Pain and Posthuman Life Writing." *Biography* 35, no. 1 (2012): 83–98.

Gingrich-Philbrook, Craig. "Evaluating (Evaluations of) Autoethnography." In *Handbook of Autoethnography*, edited by Stacy Holman Jones, Tony E. Adams, and Carolyn Ellis, 609–26. 2013. Routledge London, 2016.

Globalization Partners. "Indonesia—Employer of Record." Globalization Partners website. Last accessed March 23, 2022. www.globalization-partners.com.

Golash-Boza, Tanya. *Race and Racisms*. 2nd ed. Oxford University Press, 2015.

Goodeve, Thyrza Nichols. "You Sober People." In *When Pain Strikes*, edited by Bill Burns, Cathy Busby, and Kim Sawchuk, 228–47. University of Minnesota Press, 1999.

Graham-McLay, Charlotte. "Under Pressure, New Zealand Ends a Refugee Policy Branded Racist." *New York Times*, October 4, 2019. www.nytimes.com.

Grewal, Inderpal. *Home and Harem: Nation, Gender, Empire, and the Cultures of Travel*. Duke University Press, 1996.

Grewal, Inderpal, and Caren Kaplan. "Global Identities: Theorizing Transnational Studies of Sexuality." In *Feminist and Queer Theory*, edited by L. Ayu Saraswati and Barbara Shaw, 47–57. Oxford University Press, 2020.

Gudmannsdottir, Gudrun, and Sigridur Halldorsdottir. "Primacy of Existential Pain and Suffering in Residents in Chronic Pain in Nursing Homes: A Phenomenological Study." *Scandinavian Journal of Caring Sciences* 23 (2009): 317–27.

Guerin, Bernard. "Replacing Catharsis and Uncertainty Reduction Theories with Descriptions of Historical and Social Context." *Review of General Psychology* 5 (2001): 44–61.

Gunning, Isabelle R. "Arrogant Perception, World-Travelling, and Multicultural Feminism: The Case of Female Genital Surgeries." *Columbia Human Rights Law Review* 23, no. 2 (1992): 189–248.

Halberstam, Judith. *The Queer Art of Failure.* Duke University Press, 2011.

Ham, Julie, and Merina Sunuwar. "Experiments in Enchantment: Domestic Workers, Upcycling, and Social Change." *Emotion, Space and Society* 37 (2020): 1–9.

Harding, Jennifer, and E. Deidre Pribram. "Losing Our Cool? Following Williams and Grossberg on Emotions." *Cultural Studies* 18, no. 6 (2004): 863–83.

Heleniak, Timothy, and Hjördis Rut Sigurjonsdottir. "Once Homogenous, Tiny Iceland Opens Its Doors to Immigrants." Migration Policy Institute, April 18, 2018. www.migrationpolicy.org.

Hemmings, Clare. *Why Stories Matter: The Political Grammar of Feminist Theory.* Duke University Press, 2011.

Hide, Louise, Joanna Bourke, and Carmen Mangion. "Introduction: Perspectives on Pain." *19: Interdisciplinary Studies in the Long Nineteenth Century* 15 (2012), https://doi.org/10.16995/ntn.663.

Holland, Patrick, and Graham Huggan. *Tourists with Typewriters: Critical Reflections on Contemporary Travel Writing.* University of Michigan Press, 1998.

Hood, Erin. "Re-Articulating Physical Pain through Artistic Performance, Performance as a Mode of Analysis, and Performance-Making." PhD diss., University of Wisconsin–Madison, 2013.

hooks, bell. *Feminist Theory: From Margin to Center.* 1984. Routledge, 2014.

———. *Yearning: Race, Gender, and Cultural Politics.* South End Press, 1990.

Huffington, Arianna. "Politics Is Making America Sick: A Guide for Staying Healthy as We Go into the 2020 Election." *Thrive,* October 2, 2019. https://thriveglobal.com.

Humas. "Per 1 Mei 2020 Iuran Peserta Segmen PBPU dan BP Telah Disesuaikan." BPJS Kesehatan, April 30, 2020. https://bpjs-kesehatan.go.id.

Iceland Review. "In Focus: Mental Health Care System Criticized." *Iceland Review,* September 2, 2017. www.icelandreview.com.

Insight Meditation South Bay. "Five Aggregates." Insight Meditation South Bay website. Last accessed March 23, 2022. www.imsb.org.

Ismael, Jacqueline, and Shereen Ismael. "Between Iraq and a Hard Place: Iraqis in Diaspora." In *Muslim Diaspora in the West: Negotiating Gender, Home, and Belonging,* edited by Haideh Moghissi and Halleh Ghorashi, 197–208. Ashgate, 2010.

Jackson, Michael. *Paths toward a Clearing: Radical Empiricism and Ethnographic Inquiry.* Indiana University Press, 1989.

June-Rodgers, Pamela. "Bodily and Narrative Fragmentation: Wounds, Scars, and Feminist Healing in Selected Novels by Postmodern Multiethnic American Women." PhD diss., Indiana University of Pennsylvania, 2009.

Juschka, Darlene. "Pain, Gender, and Systems of Belief and Practice." *Religion Compass* 5, no.1, (2011): 708–19.

Jussawalla, Feroza. "South Asian Diaspora Writers in Britain: 'Home' versus 'Hybridity.'" In *Ideas of Home: Literature of Asian Migration*, edited by Geoffrey Kain, 17–37. Michigan State University, 1997.

Kabir, Ananya. "Double Violation? (Not) Talking about Sexual Violence in Contemporary South Asia." In *Feminism, Literature, and Rape Narratives: Violence and Violation*, edited by Sorcha Gunne and Zoe Thompson, 146–63. Routledge, 2012.

Kaplan, Caren. "Hillary Rodham Clinton's Orient: Cosmopolitan Travel and Global Feminist Subjects." *Meridians* 2, no. 1 (2001): 219–40.

———. *Questions of Travel: Postmodern Discourses of Displacement*. Duke University Press, 1996.

Katz, James D. "Pain Does Not Suffer Misprision: An Inquiry into the Presence and Absence That Is Pain." *Medical Humanities* 30, no. 2 (2004): 59–62.

Kearney, Richard. "Narrating Pain: The Power of Catharsis." *Paragraph* 30, no. 1 (2007): 51–66.

Keating, Analouise, and Kakali Bhattacharya. "Decolonizing Religion, Transforming Spirit: The Imaginal in Gloria Anzaldúa's Autohistoria-Teoría." In *Feminist and Queer Theory*, edited by L. Ayu Saraswati and Barbara Shaw, 523–38. Oxford University Press, 2020.

Keating, Christine. "Framing the Postcolonial Sexual Contract: Democracy, Fraternalism, and State Authority in India." *Hypatia* 22, no. 4 (2007): 130–45.

Kelleher, Suzanne. "This Is Your Brain on Travel." *Forbes*, July 28, 2019. www.forbes.com.

Kelley, Joyce. *Excursions into Modernism: Women Writers, Travel, and the Body*. Ashgate, 2015.

Kharisma, Dewi. "3 Hal Yang Perlu Kamu Tahu Sebelum Pindah Kelas BPJS Kesehatan." PLuang, December 1, 2019. https://blog.pluang.com.

Khattak, Saba. "Violence and Home: Afghan Women's Experience of Displacement." In *Gender, Conflict, and Migration*, edited by Navnita Behera, 116–36. Sage, 2006.

Kim, Youna. "Digital Diaspora, Mobility, and Home." In *Routledge Handbook of East Asian Popular Culture*, edited by Koichi Iwabuchi et al., 55–65. Routledge, 2017.

Kinsley, Zoë. "Narrating Travel, Narrating the Self: Considering Women's Travel Writing as Life Writing." *Bulletin of the John Rylands Library* 90, no. 2 (2014): 67–84.

Kleinman, Arthur, Veena Das, and Margaret Lock, eds. "Introduction." *Social Suffering*, special issue of *Daedalus* 125, no. 1 (1996): xi–xx, edited by Arthur Kleinman, Veena Das, and Margaret Lock.

Knopp, Lisa. "Household Words." *Michigan Quarterly Review* 40, no. 4 (Fall 2001): 713–25.

Lambert, Brent. "The Bloom Effect: The Neuroscience of How Long-term Travel Rebuilds Your Brain and Personality Forever." *Feel Guide*, June 27, 2019. www.feelguide.com.

Lane, Nikki. "Bringing Flesh to Theory: Ethnography, Black Queer Theory, and Studying Black Sexualities." *Feminist Studies* 42, no. 3 (2016): 632–48.

Laura, Crystal. "Intimate Inquiry: Love as 'Data' in Qualitative Research." *Cultural Studies ↔ Critical Methodologies* 13, no. 4 (2013): 289–92, https://doi.org/10.1177/1532708613487875.

Leder, Drew. "The Experiential Paradoxes of Pain." *Journal of Medicine and Philosophy* 41 (2016): 444–60.

Leed, Eric. *The Mind of the Traveller: From Gilgamesh to Global Tourism*. Basic Books, 1991.

Leve, Michelle. "Reproductive Bodies and Bits: Exploring Dilemmas of Egg Donation under Neoliberalism." *Studies in Gender and Sexuality* 14, no. 4 (2013): 277–88.

Levine, George. *Darwin Loves You: Natural Selection and the Re-Enchantment of the World*. Princeton University Press, 2006.

Library of Congress. "Nepal: Minimum Wage Increased." Library of Congress website. Last accessed March 23, 2022. www.loc.gov.

Livingston, Gretchen, and Deja Thomas. "Among 41 Countries, only U.S. Lacks Paid Parental Leave." Pew Research, December 16, 2019. www.pewresearch.org.

Livingston, Julie. "The Social Phenomenology of the Next Epidemic: Pain and the Politics of Relief in Botswana's Cancer Ward." In *Living and Dying in the Contemporary World: A Compendium*, edited by Veena Das and Clara Han, 185–204. University of California Press, 2015.

Lorde, Audre. *Sister Outsider: Essays and Speeches*. Crossing Press, 2007. Ebook.

Lugones, María. *Pilgrimages/Peregrinajes: Theorizing Coalition against Multiple Oppressions*. Rowman & Littlefield, 2003.

Lyon, John B. "'You Can Kill, but You Cannot Bring to Life': Aesthetic Education and the Instrumentalization of Pain in Schiller and Holderlin." *Literature and Medicine* 24, no. 1 (2005): 31–50.

Lysaught, Therese. "Docile Bodies: Transnational Research Ethics as Biopolitics." *Journal of Medicine and Philosophy* 34 (2009): 384–408.

MacAllister, Lorissa, et al. "Exploring Inpatients' Experiences of Healing and Healing Spaces: A Mixed Methods Study." *Journal of Patient Experience* 3, no. 4 (2016): 119–30.

Malik, Kamran, and Fouzia Naeem Khan. "Narcissistic Leadership at Workplace and the Degree of Employee Psychological Contract: A Comparison of Public and Private Sector Organizations in Pakistan." *International Journal of Economics, Business, and Management Studies* 2, no. 3 (2013): 116–27.

Mallett, Shelley. "Understanding Home: A Critical Review of the Literature." *Sociological Review* 52, no. 1 (2004): 62–89.

Mangion, Carmen M. "'Why, Would You Have Me Live upon a Gridiron?': Pain, Identity, and Emotional Communities in Convent Culture." *19: Interdisciplinary Studies in the Long Nineteenth Century* 15 (2012), http://19.bbk.ac.uk.

Manuel, Earthlyn. "Transforming Suffering into Enchantment as a Living Praxis for African American Women: A Self-Exploration." PhD diss., California Institute for Integral Studies, 2000.

Mariskind, Clare. "Good Mothers and Responsible Citizens: Analysis of Public Support for the Extension of Paid Parental Leave." *Women's Studies International Forum* 61 (2017): 14–19.

McGlotten, Shaka. *Virtual Intimacies: Media, Affect, and Queer Sexuality*. State University of New York Press, 2013.

McRobbie, Angela. "Top Girls?" *Cultural Studies* 21, no. 4–5 (2007): 718–37.

McWeeny, Jennifer. "The Feminist Phenomenology of Excess: Ontological Multiplicity, Auto-Jealousy, and Suicide in Beauvoir's *L'Invitée*." *Continental Philosophy Review* 45 (2012): 41–75.

Merleau-Ponty, Maurice. *Phenomenology of Perception*. Routledge, 2012.

Miles, Martina. "Pain in Parallel Places: Interventions in Disability Studies and Science Fiction." PhD diss., University of Oregon, 2015.

Mills, Charles. *The Racial Contract*. Cornell University Press, 1997.

Mills, Sara. *Discourses of Difference: An Analysis of Women's Travel Writing and Colonialism*. Routledge, 1991.

Mohsen, Ali Mohamed. "Emotion as First Philosophy." PhD diss. Stony Brook University, 2018.

Moraga, Cherríe, and Gloria Anzaldúa. "Entering the Lives of Others: Theory in the Flesh." In *This Bridge Called My Back: Writings by Radical Women of Color*, 2nd ed., edited by Cherríe Moraga and Gloria Anzaldúa. New York: Kitchen Table Women of Color Press, 1983.

Moss, Joshua. "Defining Transcomedy: Humor, Tricksterism, and Postcolonial Affect from Gerald Vizenor to Sacha Baron Cohen." *International Journal of Cultural Studies* 19, no. 5 (2016): 487–500.

Moussawi, Ghassan. "Bad Feelings: On Trauma, Nonlinear Time, and Accidental Encounters in 'The Field.'" *Departures in Critical Qualitative Research* 10, no. 1 (2021): 78–96.

Mukherjee, Siddhartha. *The Emperor of All Maladies: A Biography of Cancer*. Fourth Estate, 2011.

Mulla, Sameena. *The Violence of Care: Rape Victims, Forensic Nurses, and Sexual Assault Intervention*. NYU Press, 2014.

Murray, Jessica. "A Post-Colonial and Feminist Reading of Selected Testimonies to Trauma in Post-Liberation South Africa and Zimbabwe." *Journal of African Cultural Studies* 21, no. 1 (2009): 1–21.

Naber, Nadine. "How to Name and Claim Your Theoretical Approach." Nadine Naber website, February 7, 2021. Last accessed September 10, 2021. https://nadinenaber.com.

Naraindasa, Harish, and Cristiana Bastos. "Introduction: Special Issue for Anthropology and Medicine: Healing Holidays? Itinerant Patients, Therapeutic Locales, and the Quest for Health." *Anthropology & Medicine* 18, no. 1 (2011): 1–6.

National Institute of Mental Health. "Any Anxiety Disorder." National Institute of Mental Health website. Last accessed June 12, 2022. www.nimh.nih.gov.

———. "Major Depression." National Institute of Mental Health website. Last accessed June 12, 2022. www.nimh.nih.gov.

———. "Post-Traumatic Stress Disorder (PTSD)." National Institute of Mental Health website. Last accessed March 23, 2022. www.nimh.nih.gov.

Nets-Zehngut, Rafi. "Collective Self-Healing Process: The Israeli-Palestinian Case Conflict Resolution." *Quarterly* 30, no. 2 (2012): 243–67.

Newmahr, Staci. "Power Struggles: Pain and Authenticity in SM Play." *Symbolic Interaction* 33, no. 3 (2010): 389–411.

New Scientist. "Anamorphic Art." *New Scientist*, December 4, 2008. www.newscientist.com.

New Zealand Immigration. "Live Permanently in New Zealand." New Zealand Immigration website. Last accessed April 18, 2022. www.immigration.govt.nz.

New Zealand Now. "Healthcare Services." New Zealand Now website. Last accessed April 18, 2022. www.newzealandnow.govt.nz.

———. "Paying for Healthcare Services." New Zealand Now website. Last accessed March 23, 2022. www.newzealandnow.govt.nz.

Nithitham, Diane. *Making Home in Diasporic Communities: Transnational Belonging amongst Filipina Migrants*. Routledge, 2016.

Ojala, Tapio, et al. "The Dominance of Chronic Pain: A Phenomenological Study." *Musculoskeletal Care* 12 (2014): 141–49.

Olalquiaga, Celeste. "Pain Practices and the Reconfiguration of Physical Experience." In *When Pain Strikes*, edited by Bill Burns, Cathy Busby, and Kim Sawchuk, 255–66. University of Minnesota Press, 1999.

Orlan. "Intervention." In *The Ends of Performance*, edited by Peggy Phelan and Jill Lane, 315–27. NYU Press, 1998.

Orwell, George. *A Collection of Essays*. Houghton Mifflin, 1981.

Pagis, Michal. "Embodied Self-Reflexivity." *Social Psychology Quarterly* 72, no 3 (2009): 265–83.

Paramaditha, Intan. "On the Complicated Questions around Writing about Travel." *Literary Hub*, March 2, 2020. https://lithub.com.

Pateman, Carole. *The Sexual Contract*. Polity, 1988.

Pfaelzer, Jean. "Tillie Olsen's 'Tell Me a Riddle': The Dialectics of Silence." *Frontiers: A Journal of Women Studies* 15, no. 2 (1994): 1–22.

Philipose, Liz. "The Politics of Pain and the End of Empire." *International Feminist Journal of Politics* 9, no. 1 (2007): 60–81.

Pitugshatwong, Nuntiya. "Crossing Boundaries: Domestic Fiction and Nineteenth-Century Women's Travel Narratives." PhD diss., University of Minnesota, 2008.

Potter, Brett. "Tracing the Landscape: Re-Enchantment, Play, and Spirituality in Parkour." *Religions* 10, no. 9 (2019): 505, https://doi.org/10.3390/rel10090505.

Puwar, Nirmal, and Carole Pateman. "Interview with Carole Pateman: 'The Sexual Contract,' Women in Politics, Globalization, and Citizenship." *Feminist Review* 70 (2002): 123–33.

Rahman, Ubaid Ur, et al. "Does Team Orientation Matter? Linking Work Engagement and Relational Psychological Contract with Performance." *Journal of Management Development* 36, no. 9 (2017): 1102–13.

Rajiva, Mythili. "'Better Lives': The Transgenerational Positioning of Social Mobility in the South Asian Canadian Diaspora." *Women's Studies International Forum* 36 (2013): 16–26.

Ramos, Maria. "Literary Cartographies of Spain: Mapping Identity in African American Travel Writing." PhD diss., University of Maryland, 2011.

Roberson, Susan, ed. *Defining Travel: Diverse Visions.* University Press of Mississippi, 2001.

Rodriguez, Amardo. "The Exile Narratives." In *Stories of Home: Place, Identity, Exile*, edited by Devika Chawla and Stacy Holman Jones, 105–12. Lexington Books, 2015.

Rokom. "Kemenkes Beberkan Masalah Permasalahan Kesehatan Jiwa di Indonesia." Sehat Negeriku Kementrian Kesehatan (Ministry of Health), October 7, 2021. https://sehatnegeriku.kemkes.go.id.

Rottenberg, Catherine. *The Rise of Neoliberal Feminism.* Oxford University Press, 2018.

Rousseau, Jean-Jaques. *The Social Contract.* Translated by Tom Griffith. Wordsworth Editions, 2013. Ebook.

Roy, Eleanor Ainge. "New Zealand 'Wellbeing' Budget Promises Billions to Care for Most Vulnerable." *Guardian*, May 29, 2019. www.theguardian.com.

Saadawi, Nawal el. *My Travels around the World.* Translated by Shirley Ever. Methuen London, 1991.

Said, Edward. *Orientalism.* Vintage Books, 1979.

Saraswati, L. Ayu. *Pain Generation: Social Media, Feminist Activism, and the Neoliberal Selfie.* NYU Press, 2021.

———. "Wikisexuality: Rethinking Sexuality in Cyberspace." *Sexualities* 16, no. 5/6 (2013): 587–603.

Saraswati, L. Ayu, and Barbara Shaw, eds. *Feminist and Queer Theory: An Intersectional and Transnational Reader.* Oxford University Press, 2020.

Saratchandra, Ediriweera. *Buddhist Psychology of Perception.* Ceylon University Press, 1958.

Satina, Barbara, and Francine Hultgren. "The Absent Body of Girls Made Visible: Embodiment as the Focus in Education." *Studies in Philosophy and Education* 20 (2001): 521–34.

Scarry, Elaine. *The Body in Pain: The Making and Unmaking of the World.* Oxford University Press, 1985.

Schweizer, Bernard. "Political Travelers: The Ideological Functions of English Travel Writing in the 1930s." PhD diss., Duke University, 1997.

Scott, Joan. "Experience." *Feminists Theorize the Political*, edited by Judith Butler and Joan W. Scott, 22–40. Routledge, 1992.

Sebayang, Susy K., Marty Mawarpury, and Rizanna Rosemary. "Less Than 1,000 Psychiatrists for 260 Million Indonesians." *Jakarta Post*, November 6, 2018. www.thejakartapost.com.

Siegel, Kristi. "Women's Travel and the Rhetoric of Peril: It Is Suicide to Be Abroad." *Gender, Genre, and Identity in Women's Travel Writing*, edited by Kristi Siegel, 55–72. Peter Lang, 2004.

Siegel, Susanna. *The Rationality of Perception*. Oxford University Press, 2017.

Sjúkratryggingar Íslands. "Payment Participation System." Sjúkratryggingar Íslands website. Last accessed March 23, 2022. www.sjukra.is.

Smith, Sidonie. *Moving Lives: Twentieth-Century Women's Travel Writing*. University of Minnesota Press, 2001.

Stanford, Ann Folwell. *Bodies in a Broken World: Women of Color Novelists and the Politics of Medicine*. University of North Carolina Press, 2003.

Stewart, Kathleen. "An Autoethnography of What Happens." In *Handbook of Autoethnography*, edited by Stacy Holman Jones, Tony E. Adams, and Carolyn Ellis, 659–68. 2013. Routledge London, 2016.

Stewart-Steinberg, Suzanne. "Girls Will Be Boys: Gender, Envy, and the Freudian Social Contract." *differences* 18, no. 2 (2007): 24–71.

Strayed, Cheryl. *Wild: From Lost to Found on the Pacific Crest Trail*. Knopf, 2012.

Svenaeus, Fredrik. "The Phenomenology of Chronic Pain: Embodiment and Alienation." *Continental Philosophy Review* 48 (2015): 107–22.

Taber, John. *A Hindu Critique of Buddhist Epistemology*. Routledge, 2005.

Tambe, Ashwini. "Indian Americans in the Trump Era: A Transnational Feminist Analysis." In *Feminist and Queer Theory*, edited by L. Ayu Saraswati and Barbara Shaw, 468–74. Oxford University Press, 2020.

Tauber, Yvonne, and Elisheva van der Hal. "Transformation of Perception of Trauma by Child Survivors of the Holocaust in Group Therapy." *Journal of Contemporary Psychotherapy* 27, no. 2 (1997): 157–71.

Te Kāwanatanga o Aotearoa New Zealand Government. "Getting Publicly Funded Health Services." New Zealand Government website. Last accessed June 1, 2022. www.govt.nz.

———. "Whāngai." New Zealand Government website, April 2, 2020. www.govt.nz.

Thero, Uda Eriyagama Dhammajīva Mahā. *Anattalakkhana Sutta: Teachings on the Characteristic of Non-Self*. Vipassanā Fellowship Edition, 2014.

Tikkanen, Roosa, Robin Osborn, Elias Mossialos, Ana Djordjevic, and George A. Wharton. "International Health Care System Profiles: New Zealand." Commonwealth Fund website. Last accessed April 18, 2022. https://international.commonwealthfund.org.

———. "International Health Care System Profiles: United States." Commonwealth Fund website. Last accessed April 18, 2022. https://international.commonwealthfund.org.

Tillett, Emily. "Some Americans Still Doubt Women's Emotional Suitability for Politics, according to Study." CBS News, April 16, 2019. www.cbsnews.com.

Top, Seyfi. "In the Strategic Sense: Evaluating Transactional and Relational Expectations as Reflection of Emotional Contract." *Procedia—Social and Behavioral Sciences* 99 (2013): 230–39.

Toyosaki, Satoshi, and Sandra L. Pensoneau-Conway. "Autoethnography as a Praxis of Social Justice: Three Ontological Contexts." In *Handbook of Autoethnography*, edited by Stacy Holman Jones, Tony E. Adams, and Carolyn Ellis, 557–75. 2013. Routledge London, 2016.

Tsolidis, Georgina. "Memories of Home: Family in the Diaspora." *Journal of Comparative Family Studies* 42, no. 3 (2011): 411–20.

US Citizenship and Immigration Services. "Find Help in Your Community." US Citizenship and Immigration Services website. Last accessed March 23, 2022. www.uscis.gov.

US Department of State. "U.S. Relations with Costa Rica." US Department of State website. September 15, 2021. www.state.gov.

Útlendingastofnun: The Directorate of Immigration. "Service for Immigrants." Útlendingastofnun: The Directorate of Immigration website. Last accessed June 12, 2022. http://utl.is.

Valentine, David. "'The Calculus of Pain': Violence, Anthropological Ethics, and the Category Transgender." *Ethnos* 68, no. 1 (2003): 27–48.

Vidal-Ortiz, Salvador. "On Being a White Person of Color: Using Autoethnography to Understand Puerto Ricans' Racialization." *Qualitative Sociology* 27, no. 2 (2004): 179–223.

Wall, Illan rua. "On Pain and the Sense of Human Rights." *Australian Feminist Law Journal* 29 (2008): 53–76.

Walsh, Mary. "Feminism, Adaptive Preferences, and Social Contract Theory." *Hypatia* 30, no. 4 (2015): 829–45.

Walters, Wendy. *At Home in Diaspora: Black International Writing*. University of Minnesota Press, 2005.

Weber, Max. "Science as a Vocation." *Daedalus* 87, no. 1 (1958): 111–34.

Weiss, Margot. *Techniques of Pleasure: BDSM and the Circuits of Sexuality*. Duke University Press, 2011.

Wendorf, Jessica, and Fan Yang. "Benefits of a Negative Post: Effects of Computer-Mediated Venting on Relationship Maintenance." *Computers in Human Behavior* 52 (2015): 271–77.

Williams, Bianca. *The Pursuit of Happiness: Black Women, Diasporic Dreams, and the Politics of Emotional Transnationalism*. Duke University Press, 2018.

Winet, Kristin. "Toward a Feminist Travel Perspective: Re-Thinking Tourism, Digital Media, and the 'Gaze.'" PhD diss., University of Arizona, 2015.

Winkelman, Michael, and Jill Dubisch. "Introduction: The Anthropology of Pilgrimage." *Pilgrimage and Healing*, edited by Jill Dubisch and Michael Winkelman, ix–xxxvi. University of Arizona Press, 2005.

Work in Iceland. "Maternity and Paternity Leave in Iceland." Work in Iceland website. Last accessed June 12, 2022. https://work.iceland.is.

World Economic Forum. "New Zealand Wants Its Politics to Focus on Empathy, Kindness, and Well-Being." World Economic Forum Facebook page. January 14, 2019. www.facebook.com.

World Health Organization (WHO). "Mental Health Workers Data by Country." WHO website. Last accessed May 31, 2022. https://apps.who.int.

Wyatt, Jonathan, and Tessa Wyatt. "(Be)Coming Home." In *Stories of Home: Place, Identity, Exile*, edited by Devika Chawla and Stacy Holman Jones, 31–46. Lexington Books, 2015.

Yamamoto, Traise. *Masking Selves, Making Subjects: Japanese American Women, Identity, and the Body*. University of California Press, 1999.

Young, Nikki. "'Uses of the Erotic' for Teaching Queer Studies." *Women's Studies Quarterly* 40, no. 3/4 (2012): 301–5.

Zaner, Richard. *The Context of Self: A Phenomenological Inquiry Using Medicine as a Clue*. Ohio University Press, 1981.

# INDEX

ACA. *See* Affordable Care Act
affective pain, 66–67
Affordable Care Act (ACA), 134–36
Ahmed, Sara, 6, 23, 142–43, 167n16
Alexander, M. Jacqui, 24, 77–78
alternative knowing, 89
*The Ambassadors* (Holbein), 10
anamorphic apparatus, 9–11, 161, 168n32
Anzaldúa, Gloria
  on autohistoria-teoría, 32
  Bost on, 12
  inspiration from, 23
  Moraga and, 170n8
  on pain, 4–5
  philosophy of, 143, 150
Ardern, Jacinda, 117–18, 124–27
arrogant perceptions, 43–45, 177n8, 178n11, 179n33
Asafo, Dylan, 127–28
attraction, 34–35
Australia, 158, 160
Austria, 153–54
autoethnography. *See* transnational feminist autoethnography
autohistoria-teoría, 32
autoimmune disease, 81–85

Barcelona, Spain, 93–95
Belcourt, Billy-Ray, 146
Bennett, Jane, 85–86, 96, 106–7, 186n41
Bird, Isabella, 97
bodies
  bodily remembering, 81, 93–97
  boundaries of, 10–11
  docile, 50–51

emotions in, 70
in feminism, 188n61
gibberish and, 75–79
habitual body practices, 97–98, 106–8
integrity of, 6
knowledge of, 186n28
movement of, 188n73
pain and, 2–3, 6–7, 62–63, 82–85, 167n20, 168n37
perceptions of, 18
psychosomatic pain, 83–84
race of, 173n35
without stories, 75–79
*Body in Pain* (Scarry), 168n37
Bost, Suzanne, 12, 168n25
Bourdieu, Pierre, 107–8, 187n56, 188n74
Bresin, Konrad, 65
Brown, Wendy, 166n5
Buddhism, 58
*Buddhist Psychology of Perception* (Saratchandra), 180n37
bullies, 59–60
Burlein, Ann, 92
Burns, Bill, 166n15
Busby, Cathy, 166n15

Canada, 63–64, 148
capitalism
  in culture, 23–24
  higher education in, 24–25
  neoliberalism and, 140, 155–56
  in United States, 150
Casa Batlló, 93
Castor, N. Fadeke, 138
catharsis, 65–66, 183n18

# ABOUT THE AUTHOR

L. Ayu Saraswati is an immigrant woman of color, award-winning author, and Professor of Women, Gender, and Sexuality Studies at the University of Hawaiʻi at Mānoa. She is the author of *Pain Generation: Social Media, Feminist Activism, and the Neoliberal Selfie* and *Seeing Beauty, Sensing Race in Transnational Indonesia*. She is also the coeditor of *Introduction to Women's, Gender, and Sexuality Studies* and *Feminist and Queer Theory: An Intersectional and Transnational Reader*. Her articles have appeared in *Feminist Studies, Meridians, Women's Studies International Forum, Gender, Work & Organization, Diogenes, Sexualities, Women's Studies Quarterly*, and *Feminist Formations*.